Bone Marrow Aspirate Concentrate and Expanded Stem Cell Applications in Orthopaedics

Edited by

Mohamed A. Imam

The Royal Orthopaedic Hospital Birmingham, B31 2AP, UK

Suez Canal University Hospitals, Ismailia, 41111, Egypt

&

Martyn Snow

The Royal Orthopaedic Hospital Birmingham, UK

General:

1. Any dispute or claim arising out of or in connection with this License Agreement or the Work (including non-contractual disputes or claims) will be governed by and construed in accordance with the laws of the U.A.E. as applied in the Emirate of Dubai. Each party agrees that the courts of the Emirate of Dubai shall have exclusive jurisdiction to settle any dispute or claim arising out of or in connection with this License Agreement or the Work (including non-contractual disputes or claims).
2. Your rights under this License Agreement will automatically terminate without notice and without the need for a court order if at any point you breach any terms of this License Agreement. In no event will any delay or failure by Bentham Science Publishers in enforcing your compliance with this License Agreement constitute a waiver of any of its rights.
3. You acknowledge that you have read this License Agreement, and agree to be bound by its terms and conditions. To the extent that any other terms and conditions presented on any website of Bentham Science Publishers conflict with, or are inconsistent with, the terms and conditions set out in this License Agreement, you acknowledge that the terms and conditions set out in this License Agreement shall prevail.

Bentham Science Publishers Ltd.
Executive Suite Y - 2
PO Box 7917, Saif Zone
Sharjah, U.A.E.
Email: subscriptions@benthamscience.org

**BENTHAM
SCIENCE**

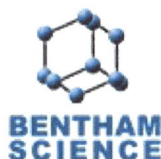

CONTENTS

FOREWORD

Advances in surgical practice have always depended upon the introduction of enabling technologies. In the mid 19th century, the introduction of anaesthesia enabled surgeons to develop procedures to remove diseased or damaged tissues. In the mid 20th century, the advent of antibiotics and greater understanding of biocompatibility issues allowed surgeons to replace damaged tissues; the introduction of immunosuppressive therapies extended this technology to transplantation of whole organs. In the latter years of the 20th century, advances in computer and imaging technologies provided the tools needed to develop endoscopic interventions. These enabled surgeons to remove diseased tissues with less collateral damage and begin to repair damaged tissues *in situ*. The 21st century has seen the nascence of stem cell technologies. Surgeons are now seeking ways to employ stem cells to regenerate damaged tissues.

At each step in this surgical journey, the enabling technologies have been exponentially more complex and sophisticated. Where surgery of the 19th and 20th centuries may have been viewed as a craft specialty, development of surgical practice in the 21st century surgery will necessitate the translation of tissue engineering, synthetic biology, materials science and computer assisted technologies into the operating environment. This can only be achieved if biologists, engineers, computer scientists and surgeons are brought together to share their skills.

Unlike genetically modified foods, the public broadly welcomes stem cell technology and patients' requests for stem cell treatments are increasing. Imam and Snow provide a much-needed insight into the development of stem cell technology and the potential role of stem cell expansion in the regeneration of damaged and deficient musculoskeletal tissues. The authors explain where stem cells come from, what makes them special, how they can be made to multiply and be influenced to differentiate into different tissues. In contrast to the public demand for stem cell treatments, legislative and governance bodies have struggled to create an ethical framework for the investigation, development and clinical introduction of stem cell treatments. The authors explain these challenges and the varying constraints on the development of this technology around the world.

Imam and Snow provide us with a snapshot of current progress in the application of stem cell expansion across the spectrum of musculoskeletal medicine. In addition to work on the use of stem cells in the treatment of non-unions and bone defects, they explore the potential for articular cartilage regeneration, repair of tendon injuries, the treatment of degenerative joint disease, revascularization of bone and regeneration of damaged nerves.

In this rapidly evolving field, Imam and Snow have provided an invaluable explanation and record of the first applications of stem cell technology in musculoskeletal healthcare. The book should prove to be a landmark in orthopaedic history and an inspiration to young scientists and surgeons alike.

Richard E Field
St George's University of London
UK
South West London Elective Orthopaedic Centre
Epsom & St Helier NHS Trust
Society for Hip Arthroscopy

PREFACE

Mesenchymal Stem Cells in the form of expanded stem cells are believed to have multipotent plasticity. The expanded stem cells are capable of being differentiated into various cell lineages such as cartilage, bone, tendon, muscle, and nerve. These unique purported properties can play a significant role in the repair and regeneration of various tissues across a number of orthopaedic specialties.

Bone marrow is regarded as the most used source of Mesenchymal Stem Cells in orthopaedic surgery and historically many surgeons have utilised unprocessed Bone Marrow Aspirate, in attempt to stimulate healing.

The main concern in using Bone Marrow Aspirate to stimulate tissue repair/regeneration is the low concentration of stem cells found within it. To address this issue, various protocols have been developed to concentrate the nucleated cell numbers to produce Bone Marrow Aspirate Concentrate.

The concept of Bone Marrow Aspirate Concentrate is to improve the recovery of the nucleated cells from the marrow aspirate, while decreasing the recovery of non-nucleated cells such as RBCs. This book aims to examine the current reported clinical applications of bone marrow aspirate concentrate and expanded stem cells and their effectiveness in orthopaedic surgery.

Mohamed A Imam
The Royal Orthopaedic Hospital
Birmingham, B31 2AP
UK
Suez Canal University Hospitals
Ismailia, 41111
Egypt

Martyn Snow
The Royal Orthopaedic Hospital
Birmingham
UK

DEDICATION

This book is dedicated to the lovely soul of my late mother; Ragaa Mohamed Ali. She was a role model in every aspect of life including science; May she rest in peace.

I dedicate it also to my father; Abdelnabi Imam for the guidance and support over the years.

Mohamed Imam

ACKNOWLEDGEMENT

I am grateful to my parents and my whole family for their priceless help and support. I am grateful to the support of my wife; Dalia, my son and best friend Yusef and my daughter Layla. I also appreciate the help from all my seniors especially Professor Field and his continuous inspiration and guidance as well as his kind acceptance to write the forward of this book. I do appreciate the eminent help from Professor Snow supervising the long process of writing this book. I do appreciate the guidance and training from all my seniors through out the years in Suez Canal University and during my different placements in the UK, Switzerland and USA.

List of Contributors

Ahmed Elgebaly	Faculty of Medicine, Al-Azhar University, Cairo, Egypt
Ahmed K. Emara	Orthopaedic Surgery Department, Ain Shams University, Cairo, Egypt
Ahmed Negida	Faculty of Medicine, Zagazig University, Egypt
Ali Narvani	Ashford and St Peter's NHS Trust, Chertsey, Surrey, UK
Amr Sami Hussien	Warwick University Hospital, Warwick, UK
Arshad Khaleel	Ashford and St Peter's NHS Trust, UK
Asmaa Kamal Abdel Maogood	Department of Clinical Pathology, Faculty of Medicine, Suez Canal University, Ismailia, Egypt
Asser A. Sallam	Department of Trauma and Orthopedic Surgery, Suez Canal University Hospitals, Ismailia, Egypt
Bassem T. Elhassan	Mayo Clinic, Rochester, Minnesota, USA
Benjamin David	Ashford and St Peter's NHS Hospital, Surrey, UK
Daniel Jackson	Queen Elizabeth Hospital, Birmingham, UK
Eman Gamal Ahmed	Department of Clinical Pharmacology, Faculty of Medicine, Suez Canal University, Ismailia, Egypt
Florian Grubhofer	Consultant Orthopaedic Surgeon, Der Balgrist University Hospital, Zurich, Switzerland
James Holton	The Royal Orthopaedic Hospital, Birmingham, UK
Kevin Newman	Ashford and St Peter's NHS Hospital, Surrey, UK
Khaled Emara	Orthopaedic Surgery Department, Ain Shams University, Cairo, Egypt
Kuen Chin	Consultant Orthopaedic Surgeon, University Hospitals Birmingham NHS Trust, Birmingham, UK
Lukas Ernstbrunner	Department of Orthopaedics, Balgrist University Hospital, University of Zurich, Forchstrasse 340, 8008 Zurich, Switzerland Department of Orthopaedics and Traumatology Paracelsus Medical University, Muellner Hauptstrasse 48, 5020, Salzburg, Austria
Mohamed A. Imam	Department of Arthroscopy, The Royal Orthopaedic Hospital, Birmingham, UK
Mohamed Mokhtar	Department of Trauma and Orthopedic Surgery, Suez Canal University Hospitals, Ismailia, Egypt
Martyn Snow	Department of Arthroscopy, The Royal Orthopaedic Hospital, Birmingham, UK
Mohamed Ahmed Mandour	De Duve Institute, University Catholique de louvain (UCL), Brussels, Belgium Department of Clinical Pathology, Faculty of Medicine, Suez Canal University, Ismailia, Egypt
Mohamed Shehata	Faculty of Medicine, Zagazig University, Egypt
Oscar Garcia Casas	Ashford and St Peter's NHS Trust, Chertsey, UK

Ramy Ahmed Diab	Orthopaedic Surgery Department, Ain Shams University, Cairo, Egypt
Rania Mohammed Kishk	Department of Microbiology and Immunology, Faculty of Medicine, Suez Canal University, Ismailia, Egypt
Rohit Gupta	Ashford and St Peter's NHS Hospital, Surrey, UK
Salma Y. Fala	Faculty of Medicine, Suez Canal University, Ismailia, Egypt
Saman Horriat	St George's Hospital, London, UK
Saqib Javid	Ashford and St Peter's NHS Trust, UK
Tomek Kowalski	The Royal Orthopaedic Hospital, Northfield, Birmingham, UK
Yasser Elsherbini	Research and Development, OxCell, OX3 8AT Oxford, UK Institute of Biomedical Engineering, University of Oxford, OX3 7DQ Oxford, UK

Introduction

Mohamed A. Imam[1,*], **Yasser Elsherbini**[2,3] and **Martyn Snow**[1]

[1] *Department of Arthroscopy, The Royal Orthopaedic Hospital, Birmingham, UK*

[2] *Research and Development, OxCell, OX3 8ATOxford, UK*

[3] *Institute of Biomedical Engineering, University of Oxford, OX3 7DQOxford, UK*

Abstract: Mesenchymal Stem Cells (MSCs) have multipotent plasticity. They demonstrate the ability to differentiate into various cell types. These include bone, tendon, cartilage, muscles and nerve [1-6]. Subsequently, they can have a role in the coming era of medicine as they have the potential to contribute to the regeneration and reconstruction of different tissues, especially in musculoskeletal medicine. As yet, Bone marrow is regarded as the most attractive source of MSCs [7, 8] and for the last few years, numerous interventionists have employed unprocessed Bone Marrow Aspirate (BMA), to incite healing.

Keywords: Bone Marrow Aspirate Concentrate (BMAC), Expanded stem cells, MSCs.

The concentration of MSCs in the marrow is known to be around 7-30 cells/million-nucleated cells [9]. To approach this matter, several etiquettes have emerged to increase the concentration of the nucleated cells to provide Bone Marrow Aspirate Concentrate (BMAC) with the aim that it would produce an adequate amount of MSCs required to produce efficacious conditions for healing and reconstruction [9, 10]. Hernigou *et al.* [11] reported that the effectiveness of BMAC depends on the concentration of progenitors cells. They examined the amount and density of these cells in BMA and BMAC taken from the iliac crest. The BMAC contained a mean of 2579 +/- 1121 compared with 612 +/- 134 cells/cm^3 in the BMA cohort. They highlighted that Diminished array of progenitor cells is significantly associated with non-union (p < 0.01).

Hyer *et al.* [12] have recommended that the iliac crest had a higher mean density of bone forming progenitor cells, especially when compared with other localities. Enormous quantities of BMA are consequently needed when aspirating from the

* **Corresponding author Mohamed A. Imam:** Department of Arthroscopy, The Royal Orthopaedic Hospital, Birmingham, UK; Tel: +44 121 685 4000; Fax: +44 121 685 4100; E-mail: Mohamed.Imam@aol.com

tibia or calcaneus to produce a comparable amount of MSCs collected from the iliac bone. Variables like age, sex, smoking, and diabetes did not correlate with the osteoblastic progenitor cell concentration [12].

Hernigou *et al.* [13] have described the sector rule for harvesting marrow from the iliac crest. This was mainly dependant on their safety zones concept. The authors analysed 480 insertion locations carried out by six surgeons in 120 cases. They recognized raised peril of breaches in overweight patients and this risk is reduced when more experienced personal undertook the procedure. They recommended that the sector rule concept is a safe way for BMA harvesting. Hernigou *et al.* [14] in another investigation further recognized that the use of 10ml syringes to harvest BMA was better than using the 50ml ones.

The chief attention in using bone marrow aspirate is the decreased quantity of stem cells attained within it, as barely 0.001% of nucleated cells are real MSCs [4, 14, 15]. Various systems have been introduced to concentrate BMA to develop BMAC. These involve the employment of Ficoll density gradients laboratories and automated systems in the clinical context. Although these systems improve the quantity of MSCs, all do not significantly improve the proportion of MSCs to nucleated cells [9, 10, 15]. Centrifugation is the modern system of preference for the numerous commercially usable commodities utilized clinically, although comparing it to Platelet-rich plasma (PRP), there is a significant disparity in the definitive end outputs achieved. Fortier *et al.* [16], examined the ingredients of PRP and BMAC (Table 1); there are decreased platelets and elevated WBC's in BMAC confirming that this is a distinct construct when compared with PRP with a distinct mechanism of action.

Table 1. Results of Cytological Analysis of Bone Marrow Aspirate and Bone Marrow Concentrate [16].

	Bone Marrow Aspirate*	Bone Marrow Concentrate*	Absolute Change*	Relative Change†	P Value
Platelet count x 103/µL	31.1	208.3	177	8.7	0.002
White blood-cell count x 103/µL	36.5	267	230	7.4	0.0007
Red blood-cell count x 103/µL)	6774	3156 -	3617	0.5	<0.0001

*These values are presented as the mean and standard deviation. N=10. †The relative change is presented as the mean with the 95% confidence interval.

The notion of BMAC is to promote the regeneration of the nucleated cells from the marrow) while reducing the restoration of non-nucleated cells (*e.g.* RBCs). The precise mechanism of action of BMAC is still not fully appreciated. Conceivably, the concentration of MSCs within BMAC will produce a primary cell origin for reconstruction of the targeted tissue. Alternatively, or in addition to, the nucleated cells may deliver various cytokines and growth factors into the delivery site to orchestrate and direct host repair [16 - 20].

This book intends to explore the contemporary published clinical applications of BMAC and expanded stem cells and its effectiveness in managing different pathologies in musculoskeletal sciences.

CONSENT FOR PUBLICATION

Not applicable.

CONFLICT OF INTEREST

The authors declare no conflict of interest, financial or otherwise.

ACKNOWLEDGEMENTS

Declared none.

REFERENCES

[1]   Baksh D, Song L, Tuan RS. Adult mesenchymal stem cells: characterization, differentiation, and application in cell and gene therapy. J Cell Mol Med 2004; 8(3): 301-16.
[http://dx.doi.org/10.1111/j.1582-4934.2004.tb00320.x] [PMID: 15491506]

[2]   Gulotta LV, Kovacevic D, Ehteshami JR, Dagher E, Packer JD, Rodeo SA. Application of bone marrow-derived mesenchymal stem cells in a rotator cuff repair model. Am J Sports Med 2009; 37(11): 2126-33.
[http://dx.doi.org/10.1177/0363546509339582] [PMID: 19684297]

[3]   Nejadnik H, Hui JH, Feng Choong EP, Tai BC, Lee EH. Autologous bone marrow-derived mesenchymal stem cells *versus* autologous chondrocyte implantation: an observational cohort study. Am J Sports Med 2010; 38(6): 1110-6.
[http://dx.doi.org/10.1177/0363546509359067] [PMID: 20392971]

[4]   Brazelton TR, Rossi FM, Keshet GI, Blau HM. From marrow to brain: expression of neuronal phenotypes in adult mice. Science 2000; 290(5497): 1775-9.
[http://dx.doi.org/10.1126/science.290.5497.1775] [PMID: 11099418]

[5]   Bruder SP, Jaiswal N, Haynesworth SE. Growth kinetics, self-renewal, and the osteogenic potential of purified human mesenchymal stem cells during extensive subcultivation and following cryopreservation. J Cell Biochem 1997; 64(2): 278-94.
[http://dx.doi.org/10.1002/(SICI)1097-4644(199702)64:2<278::AID-JCB11>3.0.CO;2-F]   [PMID: 9027588]

[6]   Kopen GC, Prockop DJ, Phinney DG. Marrow stromal cells migrate throughout forebrain and cerebellum, and they differentiate into astrocytes after injection into neonatal mouse brains. Proc Natl Acad Sci USA 1999; 96(19): 10711-6.

[http://dx.doi.org/10.1073/pnas.96.19.10711] [PMID: 10485891]

[7]   Xie A, Nie L, Shen G, *et al.* The application of autologous plateletrich plasma gel in cartilage regeneration. Mol Med Rep 2014; 10(3): 1642-8.

[8]   Majumdar MK, Thiede MA, Mosca JD, Moorman M, Gerson SL. Phenotypic and functional comparison of cultures of marrow-derived mesenchymal stem cells (MSCs) and stromal cells. J Cell Physiol 1998; 176(1): 57-66.
[http://dx.doi.org/10.1002/(SICI)1097-4652(199807)176:1<57::AID-JCP7>3.0.CO;2-7]   [PMID: 9618145]

[9]   Hernigou P, Poignard A, Beaujean F, Rouard H. Percutaneous autologous bone-marrow grafting for nonunions; Influence of the number and concentration of progenitor cells. JBJS (AM) 2005; 87(7): 1430-7.
[http://dx.doi.org/10.2106/00004623-200507000-00003]

[10]   Pittenger MF, Mackay AM, Beck SC, *et al.* Multilineage potential of adult human mesenchymal stem cells. Science 1999; 284(5411): 143-7.

[11]   Hernigou P, Mathieu G, Poignard A, Manicom O, Beaujean F, Rouard H. Percutaneous autologous bone-marrow grafting for nonunions. Surgical technique. JBJS (AM) 2006; 88(Suppl 1 Pt 2): 322-7.
[http://dx.doi.org/10.2106/00004623-200609001-00015]

[12]   Hyer CF, Berlet GC, Bussewitz BW, Hankins T, Ziegler HL, Philbin TM. Quantitative assessment of the yield of osteoblastic connective tissue progenitors in bone marrow aspirate from the iliac crest, tibia, and calcaneus. JBJS (AM) 2013; 95(14): 1312-6.
[http://dx.doi.org/10.2106/JBJS.L.01529]

[13]   Hernigou J, Picard L, Alves A, Silvera J, Homma Y, Hernigou P. Understanding bone safety zones during bone marrow aspiration from the iliac crest: the sector rule. Int Orthop 2014; 38(11): 2377-84.
[http://dx.doi.org/10.1007/s00264-014-2343-9] [PMID: 24793788]

[14]   Hernigou P, Homma Y, Flouzat Lachaniette CH, *et al.* Benefits of small volume and small syringe for bone marrow aspirations of mesenchymal stem cells. Int Orthop 2013; 37(11): 2279-87.

[15]   Kasten P, Beyen I, Egermann M, *et al.* Instant stem cell therapy: characterization and concentration of human mesenchymal stem cells *in vitro.* Eur Cell Mater 2008; 16: 47-55.
[http://dx.doi.org/10.22203/eCM.v016a06] [PMID: 18946860]

[16]   Fortier LA, Potter HG, Rickey EJ, *et al.* Concentrated bone marrow aspirate improves full-thickness cartilage repair compared with microfracture in the equine model. JBJS (AM) 2010; 92(10): 1927-37.
[http://dx.doi.org/10.2106/JBJS.I.01284]

[17]   Lee DH, Ryu KJ, Kim JW, Kang KC, Choi YR. Bone marrow aspirate concentrate and platelet-rich plasma enhanced bone healing in distraction osteogenesis of the tibia. Clin Orthop Relat Res 2014; 472(12): 3789-97.
[http://dx.doi.org/10.1007/s11999-014-3548-3] [PMID: 24599650]

[18]   Jäger M, Jelinek EM, Wess KM, *et al.* Bone marrow concentrate: a novel strategy for bone defect treatment. Curr Stem Cell Res Ther 2009; 4(1): 34-43.

[19]   Muschler GF, Nitto H, Matsukura Y, *et al.* Spine fusion using cell matrix composites enriched in bone marrow-derived cells. Clin Orthop Relat Res 2003; 2(407): 102-18.
[http://dx.doi.org/10.1097/00003086-200302000-00018]

[20]   McCarrel T, Fortier L. Temporal growth factor release from platelet-rich plasma, trehalose lyophilized platelets, and bone marrow aspirate and their effect on tendon and ligament gene expression. J Orthop Res 2009; 27(8): 1033-42.
[http://dx.doi.org/10.1002/jor.20853] [PMID: 19170097]

CHAPTER 2

Basic Sciences Behind BMAC and Expanded Stem Cells

Mohamed Ahmed Mandour[1,2,*], **Asmaa Kamal Abdel Maogood**[2], **Eman Gamal Ahmed**[3] and **Rania Mohammed Kishk**[4]

[1] *De Duve institute, University Catholique de louvain (UCL), Brussels, Belgium*

[2] *Department of Clinical Pathology, Faculty of Medicine, Suez Canal University, Ismailia, Egypt*

[3] *Department of Clinical Pharmacology, Faculty of Medicine, Suez Canal University, Ismailia, Egypt*

[4] *Department of Microbiology and Immunology, Faculty of Medicine, Suez Canal University, Ismailia, Egypt*

Abstract: Bone Marrow (BM) is a major hematopoietic organ in the human body being the main primary lymphoid organ; it is the source of production of all blood lineages. These cells are produced through an interaction between BM hematopoietic cells and the surrounding microenvironment in a unit called the stem cell niche that involves several cytokines, growth factors and transcriptional factors. The following chapter will entail an overview of MSCs, their isolation and clinical application.

Keywords: Basic Science, Bone Marrow Aspirate, Bone Marrow Aspirate Concentrate (BMAC), Expanded stem cells, MSCs, Stem cell differentiation.

BONE MARROW STRUCTURE

Bone marrow, as one of the largest body organs, is formed in the medulla of the axial and long bones such as vertebrae, femur, sternum, tibia and iliac bone. It comprises of hematopoietic tissue islands and adipose cells surrounded by vascular sinuses scattered within a meshwork of trabecular bone. Through interaction of blood-borne hematopoietic stem cells (HSCs) with a local stroma of mesenchymal lineage established during ossification, bone marrow is permanently produced [1].

---

* **Corresponding author Mohamed Ahmed Mandour:** De Duve institute, University Catholique de louvain (UCL), Brussels, Belgium; Department of Clinical Pathology, Faculty of medicine, Suez Canal University, Ismailia, Egypt; Tel: +201000737003, +32471960650; E-mail: m.fouad452006@yahoo.com

COMPONENTS OF THE BONE MARROW

Traditionally, the cellular composition of bone marrow aspirate has been studied using light microscopy [2]. Analysis of small volumes (0.1-0.2mls) revealed that neutrophils and erythroblasts comprised the largest percentage although there was significant gender variation. Neutrophils were higher in females 37.4% compared to 32.7% in males whereas; the contrary was true for erythroblasts being greater to 28.1% in males compared to 22.5% in females, which might explain the differences in adult haemoglobin concentrations.

The other components included lymphocytes 13.1%, eosinophils 2.2%, blast cells 1.4 (immature white blood cells), monocytes 1.3% and basophils 0.1%. These findings were further confirmed by the analysis of larger aspirate volumes (0.5 ml) by Yamamura *et al.* using laser photometry [3]. Despite the various used mechanisms of cellular analysis, generally, the percentages of cellular components were largely alike.

BONE MARROW COLLECTION FOR CLINICAL APPLICATIONS

There are multiple potential areas for bone marrow harvest, such as the iliac crest, tibia and calcaneus. These common areas were compared and assessed for the number of osteoblastic connective tissue progenitor cells by Hyer *et al.* [4]. The iliac crest yielded a higher mean concentration of osteoblastic progenitor cells compared to the tibia and calcaneus. This means that, higher volumes of BMA are needed in case of collection from the tibia or calcaneus to reach a comparable yield of MSCs obtained from the iliac crest [5]. Aging is accompanied with a reduction of the colony forming units (CFU-F) and consequently progenitor stem cells. Similarly, the efficacy of stem cells decreases with age [4]. It was shown that the higher the volume of bone marrow aspirate (from any accessible site including the spine), the lower the number of both nucleated cells and osteoblast progenitor cells [6 - 8]. This effect is explained by the diluting effect of blood in the subsequent samples, decreasing the concentration of colony forming units/stem cells and progenitor cells.

For a safe bone marrow aspirate, Hernigou *et al.* defined the sector rule for bone marrow aspiration from the iliac crest [9]. Computed tomography was used to examine 48 iliac crests in 24 pelvises. Then the iliac crest was divided into six equal sectors from anterior to posterior direction. Then 480 trocar entry points undertaken by 6 surgeons in 120 patients were studied and compared. The risk increased on obese patients and in the thinner sectors in the iliac crest. Additionally, the risk of injuring the external iliac artery increased in the four most anterior sectors (1 to 4) especially in females. On the other hand, posterior sectors were associated with increased risk of sciatic nerve and gluteal vessel injury when the trocar was inserted more than 6 cm into the posterior iliac crest. The use of 10 ml syringes to aspirate bone marrow was superior to 50 ml syringes yielding an average 300% higher progenitor cell. This was attributed to a larger negative pressure induced in the 10ml syringe, which preferentially removed bone marrow cells and reduced blood contamination [10].

MULTIPOTENTIAL MESENCHYMAL STROMAL CELLS

Multipotent mesenchymal stromal cells, known as mesenchymal stem cells (MSCs) [11] represent a rare population (0.001-0.01% nucleated cells) of adult human bone marrow cells. However, they can be also recognized in other adult tissues such as adipose tissues, muscles, periosteum, and other connective tissues [12 - 15]. Whereas in conjunction with additional cellular components, MSCs can differentiate and maintain haematopoiesis. Initially, MSCs were separated from bone marrow and primarily described as precursors for stromal cells or fibroblasts [16]. Subsequently, the multi-lineage commitment competence of these cells has been comprehensively characterized and studied. MSCs are non-hematopoietic stromal cells that are able to differentiate and develop into mesenchymal lineages, such as cartilage, muscle, fat, and bone (tissues of the musculoskeletal system) [17]. In the 1960s and 1970s the separation of stromal cells from BM was undertaken by plastic adherence [18 - 20], and the cells quantified by the number bone marrow derived colony-forming units – fibroblastoid (CFU-f) produced. Because they possess the capacity of self-renewal and proliferation; they are easily cultivated *in vitro* (Fig. **1**). Two subpopulations of MSCs have been identified; (i) small, spindle-shaped, rapidly self-renewing cells and (ii) larger, slowly renewing cells. The rapidly self-renewing subset was noted for their engraftment ability in mice; so they potentially show more hope for clinical applications [21].

The study of MSCs has in part been driven by their bio-physiological characteristics, which holds great potential applicability in the treatment regimens of different clinical diseases. MSCs possess immune-regulatory capacity, which explains why they are often used as tools in cellular therapies and immune-modulatory approaches.

CHARACTERIZATION OF MSCs

As there is no definite marker of MSCs, the Mesenchymal and Tissue Stem Cell Committee of the International Society for Cellular Therapy proposed minimal criteria to define human MSCs. First, MSCs must be plastic-adherent when maintained in standard culture conditions. Second, MSCs must express CD105, CD73 and CD90, express low levels of MHC-I and MSCs must lack expression of CD45, CD34, CD31, CD14 or CD11b, CD79α or CD19 and HLA-DR surface molecules. Third, MSCs must differentiate into osteoblasts, adipocytes and chondroblasts *in vitro* [22 - 25].

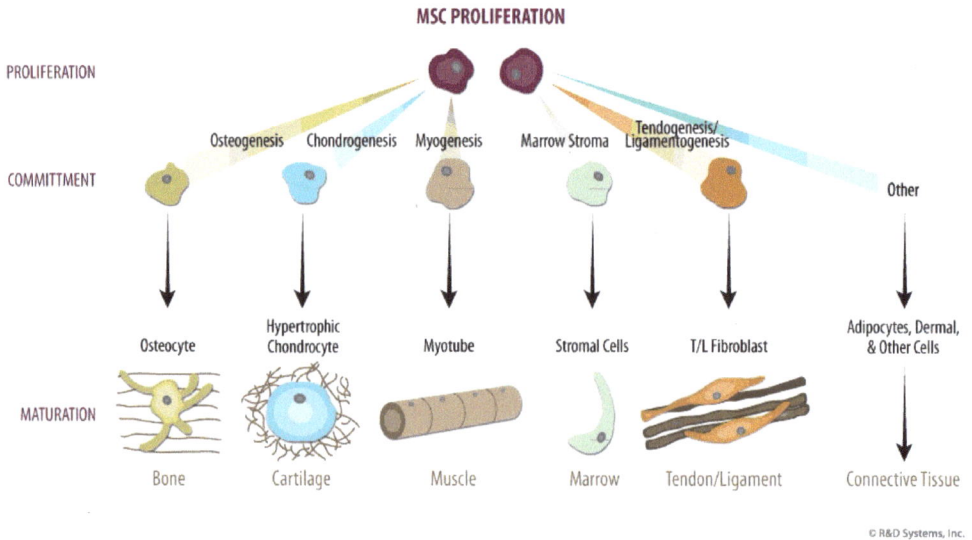

Fig. (1). Differentiation potential of MSC (Adapted after consent from R&D Systems). *

MSCs Cultivated *In Vitro* Possess Three Biological Properties that Qualify them for Use in Cellular Therapy

a. Broad potential of differentiation.
b. Secretion of trophic factors that favour tissue remodelling.
c. Immuno-regulatory properties [26].

The benefits observed in different cell therapy approaches using these progenitor cells were thought to be the result of osteogenic and myogenic differentiation. But through advances in clinical immunology, it is now well understood that, in addition to diverse mesodermal differentiation capacity, MSCs benefits arise primarily from the secretion of trophic factors and immune-regulatory capacity [27, 28].

MSCs CLINICAL APPLICATIONS

Stem cell therapy comprises the use of MSCs to replace cells and tissues damaged by congenital or degenerative disease or trauma.

In such procedures, cells are administered to patients through the blood or delivered directly to the damaged tissue of interest. MSCs are potentially applicable to many diseases, such as Graft *Versus* Host Disease following hematopoietic stem cell and renal transplant especially in the steroid resistant type, autoimmune diseases such as IDDM, SLE, RA, MS and ALS and bone, cartilage trauma and degenerative conditions such as osteoarthritis, and cardiovascular conditions as in myocardial infarction. The beneficial effects of MSCs administration regarding several of the aforementioned diseases have been analysed in animal models and phase I, II, and III clinical studies have subsequently been initiated [29, 30].

VARIABLE SOURCES OF MSCS

Bone Marrow MSCs are probably the most commonly studied MSCs, however umbilical cord blood (UCB), adipose tissue (AT), Amniotic fluid (AF), microvillus, Wharton jelly and peripheral blood as alternative sources are increasing in popularity. Other less frequent sources include: skeletal muscle, synovial membranes, dental pulp, periodontal ligaments, cervical tissue, menstrual blood, and foetal tissues such as blood, liver (Fig. **2**) [23, 24].

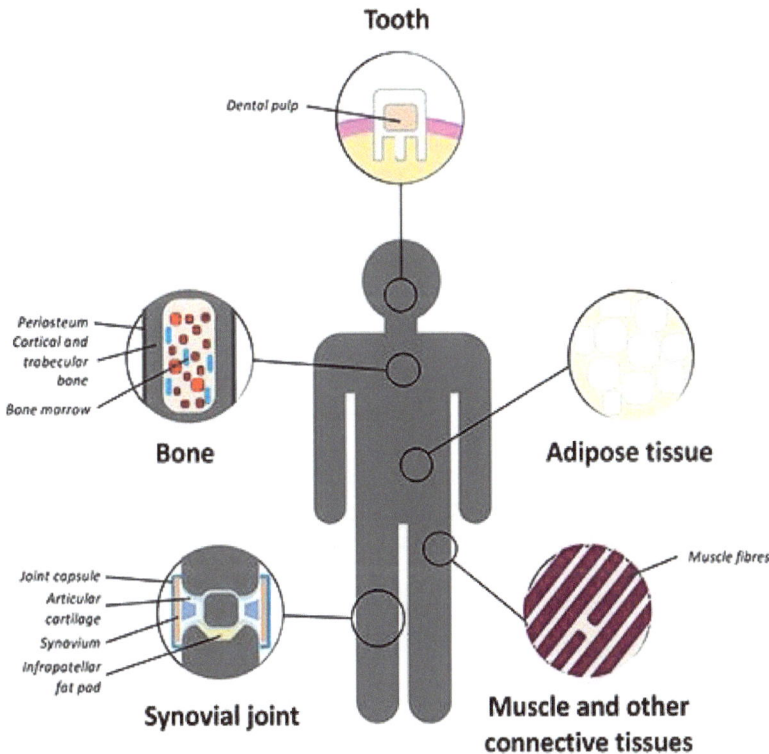

Fig. (2). Schematic representation of the main tissue reservoirs of MSCs in the human body (Adapted after consent from Fellows Christopher, *et al.* 2016).

A decision with regards to the selection of the most appropriate MSC is dependent on a number of factors. These include the ease harvest, cell isolation and expansion. An increase in age is accompanied by less available MSC's in the BM, furthermore, these cells will have a lower differentiation capacity and shorter lifespan [31 - 40]. Adipose tissue contains the highest number of MSC per unit volume while umbilical cord blood contains the youngest stem cells available [34, 35]. UCB as a source of MSC's has multiple advantages, including good longevity of therapeutic action [36]. Furthermore, UCB banks have been established worldwide to meet the technological necessities for cellular products to be used clinically [37 - 39]. On the other hand, MSCs are of low frequency in umbilical cord blood (UCB-MSC), and consistent isolation is difficult [36]. UCB-MSC has a superior proliferation and differentiation rate, beyond that of those derived from BM and AT. UCB-MSC are also much smaller in size than the other two sources [40].

UCB have shown to contain other MSC-like cells that were identified as unrestricted somatic stem cells (USSC). This nomenclature was based on their capability to differentiate into the three-germ layers and reprints a totally different distinct population compared to the CBMSC [41 - 43]. MSCs have been also found to be abundant in different fetal tissues, including liver, blood, kidney, lung and spleen [44, 45].

MSC SEPARATION

The main concept of MSC isolation from different sources is to obtain the adherent fibroblast like cell layer and subsequent processing.

BONE MARROW & UMBILICAL CORD BLOOD

Here the mononuclear cell layer is the main cellular compartment of interest. Two different systems may be used for isolation of mononuclear cells (MNC):

• A concentrating automated closed centrifugation system to separate MNC that contains the MSC for use directly in clinical setting.
• Manual laboratory open separation system using Ficoll-Hypaque.

According to the commonly used protocols, 60 ml of BM are aspirated in anti-coagulated syringe (using either citrate dextrose A or heparin) from the iliac crest from donors. Aspiration is usually performed at multiple locations around the anterior superior iliac spine in order to reduce the chance for peripheral blood contamination when more than 10 mls is aspirated at a single entry point [46].

Mononuclear cells (MNC) are first isolated from BM aspirates. After an overnight culture incubation step to allow for cell adherence, non-adherent cells are discarded (use of high concentration of FBS allow for better separation). Then the cell passage is done subsequently till obtaining mature adipocytes which are then washed and removed. MSCs are finally harvested *via* the enzymatic digestion of the extracellular matrix and then cells are seeded and cultured in the same conditions as BM [54].

The number of isolated MSCs per millilitres of native BM can be assessed by Colony forming unit (CFU) assay (Table **1**). Here, mononuclear cells are cultured at different starting densities of 5000, 25 000, 50 000 and 100 000 ([MNCs]/ml) into 96 well plates) in 5% carbon dioxide at 37°C for 6 days. MSCs are then selected by plastic adherence [58 - 60].

Table 1. Frequency of MSC from different sources (Quoted from MB Murphy *et al.* 2013).

Human tissue source of MSC	Frequency of MSCs (CFU-F/10^6 nucleated cells)	References
Bone marrow aspirate	10–83	[43, 47 - 51]
Adipose/ Lipoaspirate	205–51 000	[44, 47, 51 - 53]
Umbilical cord blood	0–0.02	[47, 48, 54, 55]
Peripheral blood	0–2[b]	[48, 55, 56]
Amniotic fluid	9.2	[57]

[b] Occurance of CFU-F in peripheral blood requires systemic treatment with GCSF.

High MSCs numbers are thought to be required for use in clinical applications, *e.g.* to promote bone healing, although this depends on different factors like the size of the defect [46, 61]. Thus competent separation and recovery of MSCs is obligatory. Characteristically, the mononuclear cell portion containing the MSCs is separated by centrifugation using a density gradient separation medium (*i.e.* Ficoll). This procedure requires a laminar airflow setting to prevent bacterial contamination. The isolated MSC's can then be expanded to yield larger numbers of cells in dedicated laboratory units. Avoiding the expansion step for isolating the MSCs would considerably lower the expense and facilitate the clinical application in hospitals that lack the essential laboratory facilities. However, while separating a sufficient number of MSCs through a concentration process alone in the operating theatre is potentially possible, it is open to debate whether this would still be considered minimal manipulation and outside to Advanced Therapeutic Medicinal product regulation [62].

MSC ISOLATION WITH COMMERCIAL BMAC SYSTEMS

In 1952, bone marrow aspirate concentrate (BMAC) was initially described as a natural expansion of the iliac crest bone graft (ICBG). A minute fraction of MSCs can be harvested *via* bone marrow aspiration. Traditionally, these MSCs were expanded through culture prior to use. More recently, the trend is to concentrate the harvest and directly implant them in one surgical procedure with minimal manipulation [46, 63, 64].

Centrifugation is the current technique of choice for the various commercially available products used in the clinical setting, despite the significant variation in the end yields. Although the number of MSCs is increased by these techniques, the ratio of stem cells to other nucleated cells does not [65 - 67].

Different systems utilize a dedicated microprocessor controlled decanting centrifuge system. Devices consist of a bench top centrifuge system and usually use up to four dual chamber disposables. Initial centrifugation phase separates the heavy red blood cells (RBCs) from the nucleated cells, platelets and plasma. Then this plasma and cellular elements are automatically shifted into the second chamber and concentrated by centrifugation. Afterwards, some of the supernatant plasma is discarded and the cellular elements are re-suspended in the remaining plasma. The starting volume utilized by each system may vary; although the average volume of bone marrow is usually between 60 – 120 mls. The whole process requires minimum operator intervention and is usually processed in less than 15 minutes, producing 6-12 mls of BMAC [66].

The principle of BMAC is to minimize the recovery of non- nucleated cells (*i.e.* RBCs) from the bone marrow aspirate, while increasing nucleated cells recovery. MSCs contained within BMAC provides a cell source for host tissues repair and the nucleated cells convey various cytokines and growth factors into the delivery site [62, 67 - 69].

BMAC has the potential to deliver a number of important growth factors *i.e.* platelet-derived growth factor (PDGF), transforming growth factor-β (TGF-β) and vascular endothelial growth factor (VEGF) [70, 71]. These growth factors are enclosed within the platelets's alpha-granules [72]. Many studies have shown that the combinations of these growth factors are critical for effective and efficient chondrogenesis [73 - 75].

BMAC COMPOSTION

Cellular composition: The cells contained within BMAC are dominantly neutrophils and erythroblasts [76]. Lymphocytes occupy 13%, eosinophils 2.2%, monocytes 1.3% and basophils 0.1% [77, 78]. BMAC contains a large number of growth factors and modulating cytokines. It is worth mentioning that the comparison between the growth factors and cytokine levels between PRP and BMAC has been extensively reviewed [16]. It was found that BMAC had 172.5x the concentration of vascular endothelial growth factor (VEGF), 78x the concentration of interleukin-8 (IL-8), 4.6x the concentration of interleukin-1beta (IL-1β), 3.4x the concentration of transforming growth factor- β2 (TGF-β2) and 1.3x the concentration of platelet derived growth factor (PDGF) [77].

PRP does not only include a high platelets level but indeed the full balance of coagulation factors and many other proteins. PRP contains various growth factors like TGF-β, vascular endothelial growth factor (VEGF), and PDGF. PRP is capable of enhancing the recruitment and proliferation of stem cells, endothelial cells which might accelerate wounds healing and some tissues regeneration processes [79].

There are studies that have reported that the mixture of BMAC and PRP would further improve the healing process in some bone defects. However, it is unclear whether only BMAC or both created this effect, as they were not evaluated separately in these studies. It is currently unclear whether the combination of these two components has synergistic effects on bone healing and regeneration [60]. More work is needed to assess this proposed synergy and its consequent clinical benefits if confirmed.

HARVEST SYSTEMS (IS THERE A DIFFERENCE?)

In routine practice, Centrifuge-based BMAC harvest systems are used to overcome the low cellularity offered by traditional aspiration systems. These centrifuge-based concentration systems collectively aim at abolition of excess plasma and mature red cell count while recapturing a fraction of nucleated cell content from both the marrow and the infiltrated peripheral blood components of the aspiration. Despite the fact that centrifuge based volume reductions have become a regular practice in many regenerative orthopaedic medicine procedures. Such systems necessitate aspirating large volumes (30-240 mL) to obtain adequate stem/progenitor cellularity for therapeutic administration. Moreover, subsets of the nucleated cells obtained from the peripheral blood component of the aspirate may in fact limit the success of procedures because peripheral blood nucleated cells (not the marrow), may stimulate an inflammatory response that can decrease the regenerative potential of the marrow-derived stem/progenitor cells. Efforts are now undertaken to overcome such predicament [80].

Many studies were done to compare the progenitor cell number and concentration in different approved BMAC harvest systems. Various systems are currently available for BMAC harvest, each of which differs in the technical steps as filter use, anticoagulant incorporation and further technical procedures. The main cornerstones in these studies were: Nucleated cells (million/ml), CFU-f/million nucleated cell, Absolute CFU-f count, CFU-f/ml. These systems comprise different methods of marrow processing and centrifugation and consequently different efficacy of the concentrate, which can impact the clinical outcome of these procedures.

The technical procedures and modifications like filter use before centrifugation intend to remove fibrin, clots and debris so as to augment the availability of the CFU-f in the concentrate. Moreover, addition of heparin in addition to anti citrate dextrose (as an anticoagulant solution) inhibits CFU-f binding to the surface syringes and transfer bags and may also stimulate CFU-f formation. A positive association has been found between the number and concentration of osteoprogenitor cells delivered in autologous bone marrow grafting procedures and the clinical efficiency of these therapeutic procedures. Furthermore, higher osteoprogenitor cell concentrations (as measured by CFU-f counts) reduce the time needed to obtain union [81 - 84]. From the approved commercially available BMAC systems, the harvest system usually yielded a greater progenitor cells' number and concentration after centrifugation when compared with other systems (*i.e.* the Biomet and Arteriocyte systems) and, thus, would offer increased osteogenic and chondrogenic healing capacity [82, 85].

CONCLUSION

In the end, the potential ability of MSCs in BMAC to self-renew, expand and differentiate into different musculoskeletal tissues (*e.g.* osteoblasts, chondrocytes, fibroblasts, and adipocytes) is very interesting. BMAC has been recently utilized to support and promote bone formation and healing with encouraging results. There is an increasing interest in the clinical applications of BMAC in many musculoskeletal diseases with early promising results. Trauma and orthopaedic surgery have witnessed growing interest in the potential use of mesenchymal stem cells (MSCs) to trans-differentiate into different mesenchymal derived tissues. More basic scientific work is needed to explore the therapeutic action of BMAC. Furthermore, standardization of the commercial handling of BMAC is needed for a consistent yield that in turn will grant optimized and translatable results.

FIGURES

*Anissa SH.Chan, Electra Coucouvanis, Susan Tousey, Marnelle D. Andersen and Jessie HT. IMPROVED EXPANSION OF MSC WITHOUT LOSS OF DIFFERENTIATION POTENTIAL Ni. Stem Cell and Developmental Biology Department, R&D Systems, Inc., 614 McKinley Pl. NE, Minneapolis, MN, 55413.

**Fellows Christopher R., Matta Csaba, Zakany Roza, Khan Ilyas M., Mobasheri Ali. Adipose, Bone Marrow and Synovial Joint-Derived Mesenchymal Stem Cells for Cartilage Repair. Frontiers in Genetics , 2016; 7 : 213.

CONSENT FOR PUBLICATION

Not applicable.

CONFLICT OF INTEREST

The authors declare no conflict of interest, financial or otherwise.

ACKNOWLEDGEMENTS

Some opinions, findings, and conclusions or recommendations expressed in this material are those of the original author(s) and do not necessarily reflect the views of the editors and authors of this book.

REFERENCES

[1]   Travlos GS. Normal structure, function, and histology of the bone marrow. Toxicol Pathol 2006; 34(5): 548-65.
[http://dx.doi.org/10.1080/01926230600939856] [PMID: 17067943]

[2]   Bain BJ. The bone marrow aspirate of healthy subjects. Br J Haematol 1996; 94(1): 206-9.
[http://dx.doi.org/10.1046/j.1365-2141.1996.d01-1786.x] [PMID: 8757536]

[3]   Yamamura R, Yamane T, Hino M, *et al.* Possible automatic cell classification of bone marrow aspirate using the CELL-DYN 4000 automatic blood cell analyzer. J Clin Lab Anal 2002; 16(2): 86-90.
[http://dx.doi.org/10.1002/jcla.10025] [PMID: 11948797]

[4]   Hyer CF, Berlet GC, Bussewitz BW, Hankins T, Ziegler HL, Philbin TM. Quantitative assessment of the yield of osteoblastic connective tissue progenitors in bone marrow aspirate from the iliac crest, tibia, and calcaneus. J Bone Joint Surg Am 2013; 95(14): 1312-6.
[http://dx.doi.org/10.2106/JBJS.L.01529] [PMID: 23864180]

[5]   Pierini M, Di Bella C, Dozza B, *et al.* The posterior iliac crest outperforms the anterior iliac crest when obtaining mesenchymal stem cells from bone marrow. J Bone Joint Surg Am 2013; 95(12): 1101-7.
[http://dx.doi.org/10.2106/JBJS.L.00429] [PMID: 23783207]

[6]   Batinić D, Marusić M, Pavletić Z, *et al.* Relationship between differing volumes of bone marrow aspirates and their cellular composition. Bone Marrow Transplant 1990; 6(2): 103-7.
[PMID: 2207448]

[7]   Muschler GF, Boehm C, Easley K. Aspiration to obtain osteoblast progenitor cells from human bone marrow: the influence of aspiration volume. J Bone Joint Surg Am 1997; 79(11): 1699-709.
[http://dx.doi.org/10.2106/00004623-199711000-00012] [PMID: 9384430]

[8]   Hustedt JW, Jegede KA, Badrinath R, Bohl DD, Blizzard DJ, Grauer JN. Optimal aspiration volume of vertebral bone marrow for use in spinal fusion. Spine J 2013; 13(10): 1217-22.
[http://dx.doi.org/10.1016/j.spinee.2013.07.435] [PMID: 24075028]

[9]   Hernigou J, Picard L, Alves A, Silvera J, Homma Y, Hernigou P. Understanding bone safety zones during bone marrow aspiration from the iliac crest: the sector rule. Int Orthop 2014; 38(11): 2377-84.
[http://dx.doi.org/10.1007/s00264-014-2343-9] [PMID: 24793788]

[10]   Hernigou P, Homma Y, Flouzat Lachaniette CH, *et al.* Benefits of small volume and small syringe for bone marrow aspirations of mesenchymal stem cells. Int Orthop 2013; 37(11): 2279-87.
[http://dx.doi.org/10.1007/s00264-013-2017-z] [PMID: 23881064]

[11] Dominici M, Le Blanc K, Mueller I, *et al.* Minimal criteria for defining multipotent mesenchymal stromal cells. The International Society for Cellular Therapy position statement. Cytotherapy 2006; 8(4): 315-7.
[http://dx.doi.org/10.1080/14653240600855905] [PMID: 16923606]

[12] Nakahara H, Dennis JE, Bruder SP, Haynesworth SE, Lennon DP, Caplan AI. *In vitro* differentiation of bone and hypertrophic cartilage from periosteal-derived cells. Exp Cell Res 1991; 195(2): 492-503.
[http://dx.doi.org/10.1016/0014-4827(91)90401-F] [PMID: 2070830]

[13] Zuk PA, Zhu M, Mizuno H, *et al.* Multilineage cells from human adipose tissue: implications for cell-based therapies. Tissue Eng 2001; 7(2): 211-28.
[http://dx.doi.org/10.1089/107632701300062859] [PMID: 11304456]

[14] Jankowski RJ, Deasy BM, Huard J. Muscle-derived stem cells. Gene Ther 2002; 9(10): 642-7.
[http://dx.doi.org/10.1038/sj.gt.3301719] [PMID: 12032710]

[15] Young HE, Steele TA, Bray RA, *et al.* Human reserve pluripotent mesenchymal stem cells are present in the connective tissues of skeletal muscle and dermis derived from fetal, adult, and geriatric donors. Anat Rec 2001; 264(1): 51-62.
[http://dx.doi.org/10.1002/ar.1128] [PMID: 11505371]

[16] Friedenstein AJ, Chailakhjan RK, Lalykina KS. The development of fibroblast colonies in monolayer cultures of guinea-pig bone marrow and spleen cells. Cell Tissue Kinet 1970; 3(4): 393-403.
[PMID: 5523063]

[17] Murphy MB, Moncivais K, Caplan AI. Mesenchymal stem cells: environmentally responsive therapeutics for regenerative medicine Exp Mol Med 2013;15:45: e54
[http://dx.doi.org/10.1038/emm.2013.94]

[18] Friedenstein AJ, Piatetzky-Shapiro II, Petrakova KV. Osteogenesis in transplants of bone marrow cells. J Embryol Exp Morphol 1966; 16(3): 381-90.
[PMID: 5336210]

[19] Friedenstein AJ, Chailakhyan RK, Latsinik NV, Panasyuk AF, Keiliss-Borok IV. Stromal cells responsible for transferring the microenvironment of the hemopoietic tissues. Cloning *in vitro* and retransplantation *in vivo*. Transplantation 1974; 17(4): 331-40.
[http://dx.doi.org/10.1097/00007890-197404000-00001] [PMID: 4150881]

[20] Friedenstein AJ, Gorskaja JF, Kulagina NN. Fibroblast precursors in normal and irradiated mouse hematopoietic organs. Exp Hematol 1976; 4(5): 267-74.
[PMID: 976387]

[21] Lee RH, Hsu SC, Munoz J, *et al.* A subset of human rapidly self-renewing marrow stromal cells preferentially engraft in mice. Blood 2006; 107(5): 2153-61.
[http://dx.doi.org/10.1182/blood-2005-07-2701] [PMID: 16278305]

[22] Pittenger MF, Mackay AM, Beck SC, *et al.* Multilineage potential of adult human mesenchymal stem cells. Science 1999; 284(5411): 143-7.
[http://dx.doi.org/10.1126/science.284.5411.143] [PMID: 10102814]

[23] Seo BM, Miura M, Gronthos S, *et al.* Investigation of multipotent postnatal stem cells from human periodontal ligament. Lancet 2004; 364(9429): 149-55.
[http://dx.doi.org/10.1016/S0140-6736(04)16627-0] [PMID: 15246727]

[24] Montesinos JJ, Mora-García MdeL, Mayani H, *et al.* *In vitro* evidence of the presence of mesenchymal stromal cells in cervical cancer and their role in protecting cancer cells from cytotoxic T cell activity. Stem Cells Dev 2013; 22(18): 2508-19.
[http://dx.doi.org/10.1089/scd.2013.0084] [PMID: 23656504]

[25] Dominici M, Le Blanc K, Mueller I, *et al.* Minimal criteria for defining multipotent mesenchymal stromal cells. The International Society for Cellular Therapy position statement. Cytotherapy 2006; 8(4): 315-7.

[http://dx.doi.org/10.1080/14653240600855905] [PMID: 16923606]

[26] Ma S, Xie N, Li W, Yuan B, Shi Y, Wang Y. Immunobiology of mesenchymal stem cells. Cell Death Differ 2014; 21(2): 216-25.
[http://dx.doi.org/10.1038/cdd.2013.158] [PMID: 24185619]

[27] Prockop DJ, Oh JY. Mesenchymal stem/stromal cells (MSCs): role as guardians of inflammation. Mol Ther 2012; 20(1): 14-20.
[http://dx.doi.org/10.1038/mt.2011.211] [PMID: 22008910]

[28] Phinney DG, Prockop DJ. Concise review: mesenchymal stem/multipotent stromal cells: the state of transdifferentiation and modes of tissue repair--current views. Stem Cells 2007; 25(11): 2896-902.
[http://dx.doi.org/10.1634/stemcells.2007-0637] [PMID: 17901396]

[29] Keating A. Mesenchymal stromal cells: new directions. Cell Stem Cell 2012; 10(6): 709-16.
[http://dx.doi.org/10.1016/j.stem.2012.05.015] [PMID: 22704511]

[30] Dimarino AM, Caplan AI, Bonfield TL. Mesenchymal stem cells in tissue repair. Front Immunol 2013; 4: 201.
[http://dx.doi.org/10.3389/fimmu.2013.00201] [PMID: 24027567]

[31] Frassoni F, Labopin M, Bacigalupo A. Expanded mesenchymal stem cells (MSC), coinfused with HLA identical hematopoietic stem cell transplants, reduce acute and chronic graft-*versus*-host disease: a matched pair analysis. Bone Marrow Transplant 2002; 29 (Suppl. 2): 75. [abstract].
[PMID: 11840149]

[32] Le Blanc K, Rasmusson I, Sundberg B, *et al.* Treatment of severe acute graft-*versus*-host disease with third party haploidentical mesenchymal stem cells. Lancet 2004; 363(9419): 1439-41.
[http://dx.doi.org/10.1016/S0140-6736(04)16104-7] [PMID: 15121408]

[33] Bieback K, Kern S, Kocaömer A, Ferlik K, Bugert P. Comparing mesenchymal stromal cells from different human tissues: bone marrow, adipose tissue and umbilical cord blood. Biomed Mater Eng 2008; 18(1) (Suppl.): S71-6.
[PMID: 18334717]

[34] Mueller SM, Glowacki J. Age-related decline in the osteogenic potential of human bone marrow cells cultured in three-dimensional collagen sponges. J Cell Biochem 2001; 82(4): 583-90.
[http://dx.doi.org/10.1002/jcb.1174] [PMID: 11500936]

[35] Stenderup K, Justesen J, Clausen C, Kassem M. Aging is associated with decreased maximal life span and accelerated senescence of bone marrow stromal cells. Bone 2003; 33(6): 919-26.
[http://dx.doi.org/10.1016/j.bone.2003.07.005] [PMID: 14678851]

[36] Parolini O, Alviano F, Bagnara GP, Bilic G. Concise review: Isolation and characterization of cells from human term placenta: Outcome of the first international workshop on placenta derived stem cells. Stem Cells 2008;26(2): 300–11.

[37] Troyer DL, Weiss ML. Wharton's jelly-derived cells are a primitive stromal cell population. Stem Cells 2008; 26(3): 591-9.
[http://dx.doi.org/10.1634/stemcells.2007-0439] [PMID: 18065397]

[38] Wagner JE, Gluckman E. Umbilical cord blood transplantation: the first 20 years. Semin Hematol 2010; 47(1): 3-12.
[http://dx.doi.org/10.1053/j.seminhematol.2009.10.011] [PMID: 20109607]

[39] Rubinstein P. Cord blood banking for clinical transplantation. Bone Marrow Transplant 2009; 44(10): 635-42.
[http://dx.doi.org/10.1038/bmt.2009.281] [PMID: 19802017]

[40] Rubinstein P, Dobrila L, Rosenfield RE, *et al.* Processing and cryopreservation of placental/umbilical cord blood for unrelated bone marrow reconstitution. Proc Natl Acad Sci USA 1995; 92(22): 10119-22.
[http://dx.doi.org/10.1073/pnas.92.22.10119] [PMID: 7479737]

[41]　Garcia J. Allogeneic unrelated cord blood banking worldwide: an update. Transfus Apheresis Sci 2010; 42(3): 257-63.
[http://dx.doi.org/10.1016/j.transci.2010.03.010] [PMID: 20395178]

[42]　Kern S, Eichler H, Stoeve J, Klüter H, Bieback K. Comparative analysis of mesenchymal stem cells from bone marrow, umbilical cord blood, or adipose tissue. Stem Cells 2006; 24(5): 1294-301.
[http://dx.doi.org/10.1634/stemcells.2005-0342] [PMID: 16410387]

[43]　Kluth SM, Buchheiser A, Houben AP, et al. DLK-1 as a marker to distinguish unrestricted somatic stem cells and mesenchymal stromal cells in cord blood. Stem Cells Dev 2010; 19(10): 1471-83.
[http://dx.doi.org/10.1089/scd.2010.0070] [PMID: 20331358]

[44]　Kögler G, Sensken S, Airey JA, et al. A new human somatic stem cell from placental cord blood with intrinsic pluripotent differentiation potential. J Exp Med 2004; 200(2): 123-35.
[http://dx.doi.org/10.1084/jem.20040440] [PMID: 15263023]

[45]　Kögler G, Radke TF, Lefort A, et al. Cytokine production and hematopoiesis supporting activity of cord blood-derived unrestricted somatic stem cells. Exp Hematol 2005; 33(5): 573-83.
[http://dx.doi.org/10.1016/j.exphem.2005.01.012] [PMID: 15850835]

[46]　Quarto R, Mastrogiacomo M, Cancedda R, et al. Repair of large bone defects with the use of autologous bone marrow stromal cells. N Engl J Med 2001; 344(5): 385-6.
[http://dx.doi.org/10.1056/NEJM200102013440516] [PMID: 11195802]

[47]　Campagnoli C, Roberts IA, Kumar S, Bennett PR, Bellantuono I, Fisk NM. Identification of mesenchymal stem/progenitor cells in human first-trimester fetal blood, liver, and bone marrow. Blood 2001; 98(8): 2396-402.
[http://dx.doi.org/10.1182/blood.V98.8.2396] [PMID: 11588036]

[48]　in 't Anker PS, Noort WA, Scherjon SA, et al. Mesenchymal stem cells in human second-trimester bone marrow, liver, lung, and spleen exhibit a similar immunophenotype but a heterogeneous multilineage differentiation potential. Haematologica 2003; 88(8): 845-52.
[PMID: 12935972]

[49]　Haynesworth SE, Baber MA, Caplan AI. Cell surface antigens on human marrow-derived mesenchymal cells are detected by monoclonal antibodies. Bone 1992; 13(1): 69-80.
[http://dx.doi.org/10.1016/8756-3282(92)90363-2] [PMID: 1316137]

[50]　Jones E, McGonagle D. Human bone marrow mesenchymal stem cells in vivo. Rheumatology (Oxford) 2008; 47(2): 126-31.
[http://dx.doi.org/10.1093/rheumatology/kem206] [PMID: 17986482]

[51]　Jones EA, Kinsey SE, English A, et al. Isolation and characterization of bone marrow multipotential mesenchymal progenitor cells. Arthritis Rheum 2002; 46(12): 3349-60.
[http://dx.doi.org/10.1002/art.10696] [PMID: 12483742]

[52]　Jones EA, English A, Henshaw K, et al. Enumeration and phenotypic characterization of synovial fluid multipotential mesenchymal progenitor cells in inflammatory and degenerative arthritis. Arthritis Rheum 2004; 50(3): 817-27.
[http://dx.doi.org/10.1002/art.20203] [PMID: 15022324]

[53]　Wagner W, Wein F, Seckinger A, et al. Comparative characteristics of mesenchymal stem cells from human bone marrow, adipose tissue, and umbilical cord blood. Exp Hematol 2005; 33(11): 1402-16.
[http://dx.doi.org/10.1016/j.exphem.2005.07.003] [PMID: 16263424]

[54]　Ishii M, Koike C, Igarashi A, et al. Molecular markers distinguish bone marrow mesenchymal stem cells from fibroblasts. Biochem Biophys Res Commun 2005; 332(1): 297-303.
[http://dx.doi.org/10.1016/j.bbrc.2005.04.118] [PMID: 15896330]

[55]　Dominici M, Le Blanc K, Mueller I, et al. Minimal criteria for defining multipotent mesenchymal stromal cells. The International Society for Cellular Therapy position statement. Cytotherapy 2006; 8(4): 315-7.

[http://dx.doi.org/10.1080/14653240600855905] [PMID: 16923606]

[56]   Martinez C, Hofmann TJ, Marino R, Dominici M, Horwitz EM. Human bone marrow mesenchymal stromal cells express the neural ganglioside GD2: a novel surface marker for the identification of MSCs. Blood 2007; 109(10): 4245-8.
[http://dx.doi.org/10.1182/blood-2006-08-039347] [PMID: 17264296]

[57]   Jones EA, Kinsey SE, English A, *et al.* Isolation and characterization of bone marrow multipotential mesenchymal progenitor cells. Arthritis Rheum 2002; 46(12): 3349-60.
[http://dx.doi.org/10.1002/art.10696] [PMID: 12483742]

[58]   Kasten P, Beyen I, Egermann M, *et al.* Instant stem cell therapy: characterization and concentration of human mesenchymal stem cells *in vitro.* Eur Cell Mater 2008; 16: 47-55.
[http://dx.doi.org/10.22203/eCM.v016a06] [PMID: 18946860]

[59]   Sessarego N, Parodi A, Podestà M, *et al.* Multipotent mesenchymal stromal cells from amniotic fluid: solid perspectives for clinical application. Haematologica 2008; 93(3): 339-46.
[http://dx.doi.org/10.3324/haematol.11869] [PMID: 18268281]

[60]   Lee DH, Ryu KJ, Kim JW, Kang KC, Choi YR. Bone marrow aspirate concentrate and platelet-rich plasma enhanced bone healing in distraction osteogenesis of the tibia. Clin Orthop Relat Res 2014; 472(12): 3789-97.
[http://dx.doi.org/10.1007/s11999-014-3548-3] [PMID: 24599650]

[61]   Bruder SP, Kraus KH, Goldberg VM, Kadiyala S. The effect of implants loaded with autologous mesenchymal stem cells on the healing of canine segmental bone defects. J Bone Joint Surg Am 1998; 80(7): 985-96.
[http://dx.doi.org/10.2106/00004623-199807000-00007] [PMID: 9698003]

[62]   Kasten P, Beyen I, Egermann M, *et al.* Instant stem cell therapy: characterization and concentration of human mesenchymal stem cells *in vitro.* Eur Cell Mater 2008; 16: 47-55.
[http://dx.doi.org/10.22203/eCM.v016a06] [PMID: 18946860]

[63]   Ardjomandi N, Duttenhoefer F, Xavier S, Oshima T, Kuenz A, Sauerbier S. *In vivo* comparison of hard tissue regeneration with ovine mesenchymal stem cells processed with either the FICOLL method or the BMAC method. J Craniomaxillofac Surg 2015; 43(7): 1177-83.
[http://dx.doi.org/10.1016/j.jcms.2015.05.020] [PMID: 26138380]

[64]   Bieback K, Kern S, Klüter H, Eichler H. Critical parameters for the isolation of mesenchymal stem cells from umbilical cord blood. Stem Cells 2004; 22(4): 625-34.
[http://dx.doi.org/10.1634/stemcells.22-4-625] [PMID: 15277708]

[65]   Pierini M, Di Bella C, Dozza B, *et al.* The posterior iliac crest outperforms the anterior iliac crest when obtaining mesenchymal stem cells from bone marrow. J Bone Joint Surg Am 2013; 95(12): 1101-7.
[http://dx.doi.org/10.2106/JBJS.L.00429] [PMID: 23783207]

[66]   Bierman HR. Bone marrow aspiration the posterior iliac crest, an additional safe site. Calif Med 1952; 77(2): 138-9.
[PMID: 12978895]

[67]   Hernigou P, Poignard A, Beaujean F, Rouard H. Percutaneous autologous bone-marrow grafting for nonunions. Influence of the number and concentration of progenitor cells. J Bone Joint Surg Am 2005; 87(7): 1430-7.
[PMID: 15995108]

[68]   Pittenger MF, Mackay AM, Beck SC, *et al.* Multilineage potential of adult human mesenchymal stem cells. Science 1999; 284(5411): 143-7.
[http://dx.doi.org/10.1126/science.284.5411.143] [PMID: 10102814]

[69]   Hermann PC, Huber SL, Herrler T, *et al.* Concentration of bone marrow total nucleated cells by a point-of-care device provides a high yield and preserves their functional activity. Cell Transplant 2008; 16(10): 1059-69.

[http://dx.doi.org/10.3727/000000007783472363] [PMID: 18351022]

[70]   Lee DH, Ryu KJ, Kim JW, Kang KC, Choi YR. Bone marrow aspirate concentrate and platelet-rich plasma enhanced bone healing in distraction osteogenesis of the tibia. Clin Orthop Relat Res 2014; 472(12): 3789-97.
[http://dx.doi.org/10.1007/s11999-014-3548-3] [PMID: 24599650]

[71]   Jäger M, Jelinek EM, Wess KM, *et al.* Bone marrow concentrate: a novel strategy for bone defect treatment. Curr Stem Cell Res Ther 2009; 4(1): 34-43.
[http://dx.doi.org/10.2174/157488809787169039] [PMID: 19149628]

[72]   Muschler GF, Nitto H, Matsukura Y, *et al.* Spine fusion using cell matrix composites enriched in bone marrow-derived cells. Clin Orthop Relat Res 2003; (407): 102-18.
[http://dx.doi.org/10.1097/00003086-200302000-00018] [PMID: 12567137]

[73]   McCarrel T, Fortier L. Temporal growth factor release from platelet-rich plasma, trehalose lyophilized platelets, and bone marrow aspirate and their effect on tendon and ligament gene expression. J Orthop Res 2009; 27(8): 1033-42.
[http://dx.doi.org/10.1002/jor.20853] [PMID: 19170097]

[74]   Schnabel LV, Mohammed HO, Miller BJ, *et al.* Platelet rich plasma (PRP) enhances anabolic gene expression patterns in flexor digitorum superficialis tendons. J Orthop Res 2007; 25(2): 230-40.
[http://dx.doi.org/10.1002/jor.20278] [PMID: 17106885]

[75]   McCarrel T, Fortier L. Temporal growth factor release from platelet-rich plasma, trehalose lyophilized platelets, and bone marrow aspirate and their effect on tendon and ligament gene expression. J Orthop Res 2009; 27(8): 1033-42.
[http://dx.doi.org/10.1002/jor.20853] [PMID: 19170097]

[76]   Bain BJ. The bone marrow aspirate of healthy subjects. Br J Haematol 1996; 94(1): 206-9.

[77]   Cassano JM, Kennedy JG, Ross KA, *et al.* Bone marrow concentrate and platelet-rich plasma differ in cell distribution and interleukin 1 receptor antagonist protein concentration. Knee Surg Sports Traumatol Arthrosc 2016.
[PMID: 26831858]

[78]   Oh JH, Kim W, Park KU, Roh YH. Comparison of the cellular composition and cytokine-release kinetics of various platelet-rich plasma preparations. Am J Sports Med 2015; 43(12): 3062-70.
[http://dx.doi.org/10.1177/0363546515608481] [PMID: 26473014]

[79]   Marx RE. Platelet-rich plasma (PRP): what is PRP and what is not PRP? Implant Dent 2001; 10(4): 225-8.
[http://dx.doi.org/10.1097/00008505-200110000-00002] [PMID: 11813662]

[80]   Ng CP, Sharif AR, Heath DE, *et al.* Enhanced *ex vivo* expansion of adult mesenchymal stem cells by fetal mesenchymal stem cell ECM. Biomaterials 2014; 35(13): 4046-57.

[81]   Hernigou P, Poignard A, Beaujean F, Rouard H. Percutaneous autologous bone-marrow grafting for nonunions. Influence of the number and concentration of progenitor cells. J Bone Joint Surg Am 2005; 87(7): 1430-7.
[PMID: 15995108]

[82]   Hegde V, Shonuga O, Ellis S, *et al.* A prospective comparison of 3 approved systems for autologous bone marrow concentration demonstrated nonequivalency in progenitor cell number and concentration. J Orthop Trauma 2014; 28(10): 591-8.
[http://dx.doi.org/10.1097/BOT.0000000000000113] [PMID: 24694554]

[83]   Pettine KA, Murphy MB, Suzuki RK, Sand TT. Percutaneous injection of autologous bone marrow concentrate cells significantly reduces lumbar discogenic pain through 12 months. Stem Cells 2015; 33(1): 146-56.

[84]   Hernigou P, Flouzat Lachaniette CH, Delambre J, *et al.* Biologic augmentation of rotator cuff repair with mesenchymal stem cells during arthroscopy improves healing and prevents further tears: a case-

controlled study. Int Orthop 2014; 38(9): 1811-8.
[http://dx.doi.org/10.1007/s00264-014-2391-1] [PMID: 24913770]

[85]   Dragoo JL, Braun HJ, Durham JL, *et al.* Comparison of the acute inflammatory response of two commercial platelet-rich plasma systems in healthy rabbit tendons. Am J Sports Med 2012; 40(6): 1274-81.
[http://dx.doi.org/10.1177/0363546512442334] [PMID: 22495144]

CHAPTER 3

Ethics in the Clinical Use and Research of Stem Cells and BMAC

Ahmed Negida[1,*], Ahmed Elgebaly[2], Daniel Jackson[2] and **Mohamed A. Imam[2]**

[1] *Faculty of Medicine, Zagazig University, Zagazig, El-Sharkia, 44519 Egypt*

[2] *The Royal Orthopaedic Hospital, Birmingham, B31 2AP, UK. Suez Canal University Hospitals, Ismailia, Egypt*

Abstract: Stem cell research is rapidly progressing especially in the field of orthopaedic surgery. The processes of stem cell extraction, expansion, injection, evaluation in preclinical studies and translation into human trials are challenging. Due to the novelty and complexity of stem cell techniques, several methodological and ethical issues need to be explored. Assessment of risk *versus* benefit proportionality, selecting appropriate participants and determining a reliable therapeutic end point are major challenges for stem cell trials in humans.

In this chapter, we are discussing ethical and methodological challenges in the clinical use and research of stem cells and Bone Marrow Aspirate Cells.

Keywords: Bone Marrow, Bone Marrow Aspirate Concentrate (BMAC), Ethics in research, Stem Cells.

1. INTRODUCTION

The ethical framework of research activities consists of two elements: 1) fundamental principles that guide research activities and procedures and 2) the application of this guidance to research ethics on human beings. This led to the generation of laws, regulations and guidelines both at national and international levels to guarantee the beneficial effect of research on human beings [1]. The declaration of Helsinki [1964] and Belmont report [1979] established the ethical principles of medical research involving human subjects as; beneficence, equality, fidelity, consent, accuracy and avoiding misconduct.

---

* Corresponding author Ahmed S. Negida: Faculty of Medicine, Zagazig University, Zagazig, El-Sharkia, 44519 Egypt; Tel: +201125549087; E-mail: ahmed01251@medicine.zu.edu.eg

Mohamed A Imam and Martyn Snow (Eds.)

Stem cell-based therapy has emerged as a promising field that aims at regenerating damaged or diseased tissues. This field of research is developing at a tremendous rate. However, due to the complexity and novelty of stem cells, there are several social, ethical and political challenges that need to be examined. According to their source, there are two types of stem cells: embryonic stem cells (ESCs) and adult stem cells.

i. Embryonic Stem Cells (ESCs)

The ethical discourse of ESCs starts from their derivation from human embryos. ESCs derived from discarded or excess *in vitro* embryo are acceptable in many countries. There is significantly more resistance to the use of new stem cell lines from embryos created specifically for research purposes, which are centred around the 'start of life' and whether or not " the time of fertilisation represents the starting point in the life history, or ontogeny, of the individual". If life does start at fertilisation, this raises the question whether the destruction of pre-implanted human embryos -who have the potential to become a human beings- in the process of obtaining their stem cells, would be considered as unethical or 'sinful' if considering some religious views [2 - 4].

ii. Adult Stem Cells

Adult stem cells are also known as "tissue specific stem cells". As they are derived from adult tissues, they do not give rise to such a debate around their derivation like ESCs. The ethical questions around Adult stem cells are centred around risk *vs* benefit and impact on the living donor's well being [5].

iii. Stem Cells in Orthopaedics

During the past 50 years, biomaterial approaches have been widely used in orthopaedic surgery including implants for joint replacement and have shown considerable efficacy. However, drawbacks like loosening, implantation failure, the need for revision surgery and the subsequent reported poor quality outcomes promote research into stem cell-based therapy as a viable joint sparing alternative. With respect to orthopaedics, stem cell-based therapy has been proposed for spinal cord regeneration, critical bone defects, non-unions and cartilage degeneration [6 - 8].

Most of the stem cells used in orthopaedic surgery are mesenchymal stem cells (MSCs) which are derived from adult tissues rather than ESCs, which raise less ethical debate. However, this does not mean that testing MSCs in orthopaedic trials is straight forward. The process is full of ethical and methodological challenges due to the invasive nature of the stem cell transplantation and uncertainty about the long-term safety and efficacy. In this chapter, we will discuss ethical and methodological challenges in the clinical use and research of stem cells and Bone Marrow Aspirate Cells (BMAC).

2. STATUS OF EVIDENCE FROM PRECLINICAL STUDIES

Investigators should not move towards the first in-human trial without adequate preclinical evidence regarding the safety and efficacy of an intervention. For example: To run a clinical trial for bone regeneration, we should have adequate preclinical evidence that: 1) experimental models have tolerated this intervention with no major risks; and 2) bone regeneration was achieved *in vitro* with a proof of cell differentiation and mineralization.

The translation from preclinical studies is challenging. Scientific rationale for the first-in-human trial should be based on high quality well-designed studies. As far as possible, randomized double blind control studies are recommended. The type of animal used within preclinical trial should be as representable as possible. For example: a first-in-human trial on bone fracture should derive preclinical evidence from a large animal model rather than a mouse model because body weight and length of bones should be considered.

3. ASSESSMENT OF RISKS AND BENEFITS

The analysis of risk-benefit relationship is important in all phases of clinical trials. Interventions must not have any substantial harm to participants and in clinical research; the benefit should always exceed the risk. Therefore, in a stem cell trial, the potential harms should be no greater than the complications of the normal disease process. In these types situations, ethicists would consider closely the process of informed consent to justify enrolment in the study.

However, due to the novelty and complexity of stem cell interventions, it is challenging to precisely estimate a risk: benefit ratio in the first-in-human trials. Even with adequate evidence from the high quality well-designed preclinical studies, investigators should be cautious that the risks and benefits would be comparable to human experiments for the following reasons:

1. Differences in tissue morphology from human to animals
2. Differences in rate and mechanism of tissue healing
3. Differences in physical characteristics like body weight and bone length
4. Differences in type of injury; accidental injuries of humans differ from the uniform, precise injuries induced in animal models.

The role of investigators is to minimise risks and maximise benefits. Failure to achieve therapeutic end point is considered a risk because stem cell implantation is not reversible. Additional risks are the possibility of migration of stem cells and the development of tumours, albeit very small due to the common use of autologous MSCs. Autologous MSCs are self-donated, unlike allogenic MSCs and ESCs which may induce further tumours and immune responses. Hernigou *et al*. [9] and Centeno *et al*. [10] reported no neoplastic complications for patients treated with autologous bone marrow concentrate and autologous MSCs respectively.

Therefore, in orthopaedic stem cells first-in-human trials, there are two gaps of knowledge: 1) Uncertainty about the magnitude of expected risks; and 2) high possibility of unknown risks.

4. SELECTING APPROPRIATE PARTICIPANTS

Selecting appropriate participants in orthopaedic clinical trials is challenging. The indication of surgical intervention and suitability of the microenvironment for stem cells implantation varies according to the stage of the disease (Fig. **1**). Identification of early cases and the suitable time for stem cell intervention is key. Also, for patients at risk of degeneration, it will be difficult to determine whether developed complications are attributed to the stem cells inmplantaion/injection or not. In Table **1**, we compare the advantages and disadvantages of enrolling participants at different stages of a disease.

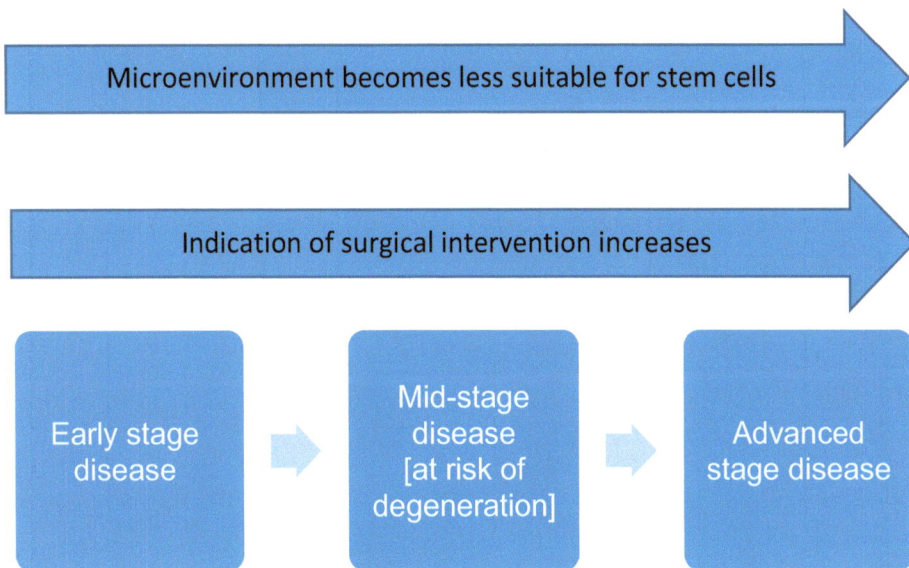

Fig. (1). The change in microenvironment and need for surgery with the progress of the disease.

Table 1. Advantages and problems with different patient populations [11 - 13].

	Advantages	Problems
Healthy subjects	Healthy participants have no serious pathology so that they are able to tolerate adverse effects.	Uncertainties and unknown risks makes it unethical to enroll healthy participants.
Patients at early stage disease	1) If the intervention is successful, they will avoid further symptomatic treatment. 2) The viable microenvironment in early-stage patients raises the chance of successful stem cell therapy.	1) It is difficult to identify early cases in some disorders. 2) Surgical interventions may not be indicated for patients with early-stage disease. Therefore, experimentation on stable cases exposes them to additional risks of undue intervention. 3) The intervention may worsen the underlying pathology and leave the patients resistant to treatment.
Patients at risk of developing degeneration	Surgical interventions are usually indicated for patients at high risk of developing degeneration, they are potentials for clinical studies.	1) The intervention may worsen the underlying pathology and leave the patient resistant to treatment. 2) It will not be clear to determine whether the complications/worsening of disease is related to the stem cell intervention or not.
Patients with advanced stage disease	1) They have less, functionally, to lose. 2) Because they do not have further therapeutic options, if they developed complications, they will undergo replacement surgery.	1) The less viable microenvironment will lower the expected benefit. 2) The advanced disease process may hinder the patient's ability to give an informed consent.

To assess the safety of a stem cell intervention in the first-in-human trial, it has been viewed as less ethical to enrol healthy subjects or patients with early stage disease. Instead, the recommendations are to enrol patients with late stage disease for whom there are no other available treatments. This is due to greater risk of losing functionality, given other known procedures. However, once the safety of a stem cell intervention has been established in phase I clinical trials, patients with early stage disease and stable patients whom are at risk of degeneration could be considered.

In stem cell clinical trials, the choice of comparator is challenging with controversial ethical and methodological issues. The aim of BMAC and stem cells injections is to regenerate damaged tissues and this novel therapeutic target is not usually achieved by any conventional treatment. Therefore, due to the novel therapeutic target, there is no standard comparator with the same target.

Since patients enrolled in clinical trials should not be deprived from a beneficial intervention, an active comparator should be provided if possible. There is a trend towards assessing the safety and efficacy of stem cells interventions with the standard care which targets slowing or preventing disease progress. Standard care is a suitable option for some conditions (*e.g.* microfracture in cartilage repair). Here, the standard care can improve the underlying condition. Although the comparison of standard care *vs.* stem cells injection will not allow blinding of the clinical trial, the ethical value has the priority over the methodological ideal. There is the potential for harm due to invasiveness of the procedure, wounds and the risk around anaesthesia. We can conclude that the use of placebo will improve the clinical trial's design and increase the scientific validity but it may be unethical to expose patients to risks of undue surgery. Minimally invasive procedures and saline injections are less of a problem ethically with regards to risk *vs* benefit.

5. STUDY DESIGN RELATED ISSUES

Determining the Outcome Measurement

Determining a therapeutic end point is another challenging issue in orthopaedic surgeries since radiographic measures do not fully correlate with the clinical symptoms of the patient. Up until now, a causative relationship between pain experience of patients and bone and/or cartilage degeneration has not been established, with psychological factors often playing a role. Therefore, it would not be appropriate to determine the treatment end point based on radiographic findings only. The radiographic findings of X-ray may indicate complete bone healing despite the patient suffering from pain or disability. An integration of clinical findings, patient symptoms, and functionality of the diseased part in the form of an outcome score should occur. A number of investigators have suggested adding physiological and metabolic markers to evaluate the homeostasis of musculoskeletal tissues as another parameter for therapeutic end point [14].

Dependent on the pathology under investigation, an appropriate length of follow-up should be undertaken. In this regard, Niemansburg *et al.* [15] discussed the challenges of enrolling patients at risk of degeneration. They recommended that studies on this type of population require longer follow up period; *e.g.* Patients with partial medial meniscectomy have a 10 to 20 fold increased risk of knee osteoarthritis. In this population, it may take years to get a radiographic evidence of developing osteoarthritis [15].

6. ADEQUATE INFORMATION AND PATIENT CONSENT

Ethical conduct of clinical research implies that patients are informed with study details and give an informed consent. Researchers should ensure that participants clearly understand the purpose of the clinical trial; investigators should provide details of study experiments, expected results, risks, and benefits. The wide translational gap between non-human and human stem cells studies and uncertainties about risks and benefits should be explained to patients. For adequate communication, graphical presentation of risk and uncertainties is recommended [16].

For stem cell research in particular, investigators should provide information as clear and precise as possible for two reasons: 1) Therapeutic misconception is common in the field of stem cells because motivated researchers and clinicians would often talk positively about it, which may be misleading to study participants; and 2) The spread of advertising websites, which trade in hope by providing information without credible scientific rationale, creates a climate of therapeutic misconception. Therefore, investigators are responsible for correcting patients' knowledge through clear and precise information supported by peer-reviewed literature.

Although patients themselves can search and read online, it will be difficult to critically appraise and evaluate the information provided online. In this regard, ISSCR guidelines for clinical translation for stem cells and the patient handbook on stem cell therapies are two recommended sources for patients to find the requisite information for clinical use of stem cells.

After patients are given clear and detailed information, they should sign a written informed consent. Informed consent is recommended also in clinical practice and clinicians should follow up their patients after transplantation to ensure their safety. Investigators can determine whether written documents are provided or not according to patients' culture.

7.   THERAPEUTIC   MISCONCEPTION   OF   STEM   CELL INTERVENTIONS

As a consistent stream of scientists, bioethicists, and politicians have praised the potential of stem cell treatment over the last decade, this has led to another problem called "Therapeutic misconception"; a term that refers to misunderstanding research goals and procedures [17]. One form of this misunderstanding is "therapeutic misestimation", in which there is an overestimation of benefits and underestimation of risk of participating in medical research [18]. Another reasons for this misconception is the language of investigators during informed consent process, often portraying hope that the intervention will be successful in treating the underlying disease.

Two major issues should be addressed to align the therapeutic misconception; 1) adequate informed consent process in which investigators should provide details of study experiments clearly to patients; 2) avoid overestimation and underestimations in scientific publications in which high public and commercial excitement can put patients at unnecessary risks, costs and unbalance the needs of desperately ill patients with the requirements of evidence-based medicine. For example: some stakeholders in ESC research announced highly promising cures for many degenerative diseases before established clinical trials which put much pressure on the field [20].

Advanced Therapy Medicinal Product

According to Medicines and Healthcare products Regulatory Agency (MHRA), an advanced therapy medicinal product (ATMP) is a medicinal product, which is either:

• A gene therapy medicinal product
• A somatic cell therapy medicinal product
• A tissue engineered product

The definition of ATMPs is found in Directive 2001/83/EC as amended by the ATMP Regulation 1394/2007 and includes combination ATMPs.

In the UK, MHRA is the competent authority:

• For clinical trial authorization for all medicinal products, including ATMPs
• For UK manufacturers or importers of ATMPs

ATMPs are new medical products based on genes (gene therapy), cells (cell therapy) and tissues (tissue engineering). These advanced therapies herald revolutionary treatments of a number of diseases or injuries, such as skin in burns victims, Alzheimer's, cancer or muscular dystrophy. They have huge potential for patients and industry.

Regulatory Protocols on Regenerative Medicines

In the UK, all regulatory enquiries about regenerative medicines should go through the MHRA Innovation Office. The Innovation Office is the single point of contact for all the regulators involved in regenerative medicines:

• The Human Tissue Authority (HTA)
• The Human Fertilisation and Embryology Authority (HFEA)
• Health Research Authority (HRA)
• MHRA

New EU and UK regulatory laws also marks the recognition that a number of advanced therapy products actually combine biological materials, such as tissues or cells, and chemical structures such as metal implants or polymer scaffolds. These combination products lie at the border of the traditional pharmaceutical area and other fields (*e.g.* medical devices). They therefore cannot be regulated as 'conventional' drugs and need adapted requirements. In addition, it should be borne in mind that a significant share of economic operators involved in this field are not large pharmaceutical companies, but rather small and medium-sized enterprises or hospitals.

8. CONFLICT OF INTEREST AND ROLE OF FUNDING SOURCE

Conflict of interest is when there is a secondary interest, quite often financial, that may affect the integrity of the research process. Evaluations of published studies showed that physicians who have financial ties with industry are more likely to report positive results than negative ones. In addition, studies funded by industry, rarely criticise their own intervention or make unfavourable conclusions. Therefore, medical journals usually ask researchers to state their conflict of interest to enable readers to recognise potential bias in medical literature.

Although, till recent time, surgical specialties were partially distant from financial interests, a study by Khan *et al.* [21] showed a strong and significant association between financial funding and reporting favourable results in orthopaedic clinical trials.

It is thought that the involvement of industry in surgery specialties was enhanced by the evolution of regenerative medicine. And it should not escape our notice that the speedy progress in stem cell research is accelerated by companies and funding agencies. This climate put researchers under pressure to rapidly introduce stem cell-based therapies towards FDA approval to get a quick return on their investments.

9. APPROVAL OF STUDIES

All clinical trials should be reviewed and approval obtained from the corresponding ethics committee or institutional review board (IRB). For multicenter studies, gaining a national approval is recommended if possible. Ethical approval is essential to ensure adherence to institutional guidelines, data confidentiality, and protection of patients' rights. Also, ethical approval is a requirement for publishing in high impact journals.

For stem cell research, because trials are ethically challenging, a detailed review of study protocols and continuous monitoring of the study process is needed. This rigorous monitoring requires that IRB reviewers to be free from conflict of interests with no ties to industry. As a result, there are some suggestions for a centralised IRB or a national stem cell ethics committee in the form of a multidisciplinary stem cell ethics committee, composed of ethicists, biologists, clinical experts and community members.

10. DISSEMINATING RESULTS TO THE SCIENTIFIC COMMUNITY

It is important to disseminate results of any clinical experiment for two reasons: 1) because it is a rapidly progressing field, there is a need to share results of new investigations to maximise the social and scientific benefit from experimental studies; and 2) due to the spread of stem cells advertising websites which provide information not supported by peer-review literature, it is important that new results are disseminated into public domain.

Withholding publication of clinical trial results creates the problem of publication bias as unpublished data may be useful for clinicians, researchers, and Evidence Based Medicine practitioners. There are many reasons behind unpublished studies: 1) researchers tend to report positive results rather than negative results; 2) journal editors are more likely to accept a manuscript reporting positive findings than another with neutral or negative results; and 3) funding companies withholding publication of clinical trials with unfavourable outcomes.

In this regard, the World Health Organisation imposed the Statement on Public Disclosure of Clinical Trial Results in April, 2015. The statement implies that 1) main findings of registered clinical trials should be submitted to a peer-reviewed journal within 12 months of study completion; 2) main findings should be published in an open access mechanism; and 3) investigators should make key outcomes publicly available to others at most within 24 months of study completion [22].

11. NON-ESTABLISHED STEM CELL PRODUCTS FOR COMMERCIAL USE

Motivated by some clinicians and researchers, patients may seek putative stem cell therapies in a "commercial market". During the restrictive policy environment of George W. Bush administration, Asian countries became a popular location for increased commercially available stem cells transplantation [23], in which many companies may lack the economic and scientific infrastructure for conducting rigorous, scientific clinical trials. Lau *et al*. [24] found that most stem cell provider websites offered therapies reported as safe, effective, and ready for routine use, which were unsupported by relevant peer-reviewed literature. There was no mention of any particular risk in 75% of the retrieved websites [24], with highly expensive costs up to $80,000 [25].

In its clinical translation guidelines ISSCR strongly condemn the demand of patients for unscientifically proven uses of stem cells or their direct derivatives [26] in addition to other guidelines and statements against the marketing of invalidated stem cell treatments for commercial gain [24, 27].

SUMMARY

The entire process of stem cell research is ethically challenging from the derivation of cells, implementing well-designed preclinical studies, translation to first-in-human trials and evaluation in the following clinical trials' phases to product lunching.

- Translation process is very challenging; researchers should precisely select adequate scientific rationale from preclinical studies. Evidence on both safety and efficacy should be obtained. Randomized, investigator blinded preclinical trials on suitable animal models are strongly recommended to narrow the translational gap.
- For the first in-human trials, patients with late-stage disease are enrolled to assess safety of the intervention. For the following phases, patients at early stage disease and those at risk of degeneration can be enrolled.
- Outcome measurement and therapeutic end point should consider organ functionality, organ homeostasis, radiographic findings, and patient symptoms all together. There is a need to develop outcome measurement that fully correlate with patient symptoms.
- If standard care can stop or slow the progress of the disease, it should be used as a comparator. Otherwise, a sham surgery will be performed while taking precautions and exerting efforts to minimize risks of sham surgery.
- All study details should be explained clearly to participants. Uncertainties about risk and benefit should be explained clearly and it is recommended to use graphical presentations.
- Researchers should avoid overestimation of the intervention either in the informed consent process or in the scientific publications.
- There is a need to develop and generalise standard guidelines for stem cell research including standardisation of the extraction, expansion and injection processes and standardisation of type and number of cells.
- Due to the rapid progress of stem cell research, there is a need to discuss and develop ethical codes to protect patients and control the process as much as possible. It is recommended that governments establish centralised, multidisciplinary and national IRBs with reviewers who are immune against financial interests.
- Stem cell research confronts two major problems: 1) the financial interest of many researchers and the increasing ties of clinicians to industry; 2) clinics and

websites, that advertise unproven stem cell products, are trading in the hope of diseased patients with no scientific rational. We fear that these two problems threaten the integrity of scientific research and will lead to diminish the trust of scientific enterprise.

CONSENT FOR PUBLICATION

Not applicable.

CONFLICT OF INTEREST

The authors declare no conflict of interest, financial or otherwise.

ACKNOWLEDGEMENTS

Declared none.

REFERENCES

[1]   Lenk C, Hoppe N, Beier K, *et al.* Human tissue research: a european perspective on the ethical and legal challenges 2011.
        [http://dx.doi.org/10.1093/acprof:oso/9780199587551.001.0001]

[2]   England MA. The developing human: clinically oriented embryology. J Anat 1989; 166: 270.
        [http://dx.doi.org/10.1136/jmg.26.9.608]

[3]   Nisbet MC. Public opinion about stem cell research and human cloning. Public Opin Q 2004; 68: 131-54.
        [http://dx.doi.org/10.1093/poq/nfh009]

[4]   Fischbach GD, Fischbach RL. Stem cells: science, policy, and ethics. J Clin Invest 2004; 114(10): 1364-70.
        [http://dx.doi.org/10.1172/JCI200423549] [PMID: 15545983]

[5]   Aalto-Setälä K, Conklin BR, Lo B. Obtaining consent for future research with induced pluripotent cells: opportunities and challenges. PLoS Biol 2009; 7(2): e42.
        [http://dx.doi.org/10.1371/journal.pbio.1000042] [PMID: 19243222]

[6]   Bambakidis NC, Theodore N, Nakaji P, *et al.* Endogenous stem cell proliferation after central nervous system injury: alternative therapeutic options. Neurosurg Focus 2005; 19(3): E1.
        [http://dx.doi.org/10.3171/foc.2005.19.3.2] [PMID: 16190599]

[7]   Magne D, Vinatier C, Julien M, Weiss P, Guicheux J. Mesenchymal stem cell therapy to rebuild cartilage. Trends Mol Med 2005; 11(11): 519-26.
        [http://dx.doi.org/10.1016/j.molmed.2005.09.002] [PMID: 16213191]

[8]   Lim J-K, Hui J, Li L, Thambyah A, Goh J, Lee EH. Enhancement of tendon graft osteointegration using mesenchymal stem cells in a rabbit model of anterior cruciate ligament reconstruction. Arthroscopy 2004; 20(9): 899-910.
        [http://dx.doi.org/10.1016/S0749-8063(04)00653-X] [PMID: 15525922]

[9]   Hernigou P, Homma Y, Flouzat-Lachaniette C-H, Poignard A, Chevallier N, Rouard H. Cancer risk is not increased in patients treated for orthopaedic diseases with autologous bone marrow cell concentrate. J Bone Joint Surg Am 2013; 95(24): 2215-21.
        [http://dx.doi.org/10.2106/JBJS.M.00261] [PMID: 24352775]

[10]   Centeno CJ, Schultz JR, Cheever M, Robinson B, Freeman M, Marasco W. Safety and complications

reporting on the re-implantation of culture-expanded mesenchymal stem cells using autologous platelet lysate technique. Curr Stem Cell Res Ther 2010; 5(1): 81-93.
[http://dx.doi.org/10.2174/157488810790442796] [PMID: 19951252]

[11] Niemansburg SL, van Delden JJ, Dhert WJ, Bredenoord AL. Regenerative medicine interventions for orthopedic disorders: ethical issues in the translation into patients. Regen Med 2013; 8(1): 65-73.
[http://dx.doi.org/10.2217/rme.12.112] [PMID: 23259806]

[12] Banja JD. Ethical considerations in stem cell research on neurologic and orthopedic conditions. PM R 2015; 7(4) (Suppl.): S66-75.
[http://dx.doi.org/10.1016/j.pmrj.2014.10.016] [PMID: 25595666]

[13] Niemansburg SL, van Delden JJM, Öner FC, Dhert WJ, Bredenoord AL. Ethical implications of regenerative medicine in orthopedics: an empirical study with surgeons and scientists in the field. Spine J 2014; 14(6): 1029-35.
[http://dx.doi.org/10.1016/j.spinee.2013.10.016] [PMID: 24184644]

[14] Dye SF. Role of technetium bone scans in orthopedic outcome evaluation. Sports Med Arthrosc Rev 2002; 10(3): 220-7.
[http://dx.doi.org/10.1097/00132585-200210030-00007]

[15] Niemansburg SL, Habets MGJL. Participant selection for preventive Regenerative Medicine trials: ethical challenges of selecting individuals at risk: Figure 1. J Med Ethics 2015; medethics – 2014–102625.

[16] Edwards A, Elwyn G, Mulley A. Explaining risks: turning numerical data into meaningful pictures. BMJ 2002; 324(7341): 827-30.
[http://dx.doi.org/10.1136/bmj.324.7341.827] [PMID: 11934777]

[17] Lidz CW, Appelbaum PS. The therapeutic misconception: problems and solutions. Med Care 2002; 40(9) (Suppl.): V55-63.
[http://dx.doi.org/10.1097/00005650-200209001-00008] [PMID: 12226586]

[18] Pentz RD, White M, Harvey RD, *et al.* Therapeutic misconception, misestimation, and optimism in participants enrolled in phase 1 trials. Cancer 2012; 118(18): 4571-8.
[http://dx.doi.org/10.1002/cncr.27397] [PMID: 22294385]

[19] Lidz CW, Appelbaum PS, Grisso T, Renaud M. Therapeutic misconception and the appreciation of risks in clinical trials. Soc Sci Med 2004; 58(9): 1689-97.
[http://dx.doi.org/10.1016/S0277-9536(03)00338-1] [PMID: 14990370]

[20] Wilson JM. Medicine. A history lesson for stem cells. Science 2009; 324(5928): 727-8.
[http://dx.doi.org/10.1126/science.1174935] [PMID: 19423804]

[21] Khan SN, Mermer MJ, Myers E, Sandhu HS. The roles of funding source, clinical trial outcome, and quality of reporting in orthopedic surgery literature. Am J Orthop 2008; 37(12): E205-12.
[PMID: 19212579]

[22] Moorthy VS, Karam G, Vannice KS, Kieny MP. Rationale for WHO's new position calling for prompt reporting and public disclosure of interventional clinical trial results. PLoS Med 2015; 12(4): e1001819.
[http://dx.doi.org/10.1371/journal.pmed.1001819] [PMID: 25874642]

[23] Friedmann T. Lessons for the stem cell discourse from the gene therapy experience. Perspect Biol Med 2005; 48(4): 585-91.
[http://dx.doi.org/10.1353/pbm.2005.0089] [PMID: 16227669]

[24] Lau D, Ogbogu U, Taylor B, Stafinski T, Menon D, Caulfield T. Stem cell clinics online: the direct-to-consumer portrayal of stem cell medicine. Cell Stem Cell 2008; 3(6): 591-4.
[http://dx.doi.org/10.1016/j.stem.2008.11.001] [PMID: 19041775]

[25] Murdoch CE, Scott CT. Stem cell tourism and the power of hope. Am J Bioeth 2010; 10(5): 16-23.
[http://dx.doi.org/10.1080/15265161003728860] [PMID: 20461637]

[26]   Society I ISSCR Guidelines for the Clinical Translation of Stem Cells Curr Protoc Stem Cell Biol 2009;Appendix 1:Appendix 1B

[27]   Qiu J. Trading on hope. Nat Biotechnol 2009; 27(9): 790-2.
        [http://dx.doi.org/10.1038/nbt0909-790] [PMID: 19741623]

CHAPTER 4

How to Design Clinical Trials of Stem Cells and BMAC in Orthopedic Surgery

Ahmed S. Negida[1,*], Salma Y. Fala[2], Mohamed A. Imam[3] and Bassem T. Elhassan[2]

[1] Faculty of Medicine, Zagazig University, Zagazig, El-Sharkia, 44519 Egypt

[2] Mayo Clinic, Rochester, USA

[3] Faculty of Medicine, Suez Canal University, Ismailia, Egypt

Abstract: Stem cells research is considered as one of the most promising technics recently. In orthopedic, the use of stem cells therapy on humans is still challenging. As a result of the novelty of these technics, the researchers need a guideline to highlight the key issues in the clinical practice of stem cells research to protect the wellbeing, safety and rights of the research subjects. Moreover, several methodological and ethical issues are still questionable regarding stem cells trials in humans as: (1) avoiding expertise Bias; (2) selecting appropriate participants; and (3) determining a reliable therapeutic end point. So, in this chapter we will highlight the key points on how to run a clinical trial and how to overcome the methodological challenges in the research of stem cells regarding orthopedic surgery.

Keywords: Bone Marrow Aspirate Concentrate (BMAC), Clinical trials, Clinical trial design, Expanded stem cells, Expertise Bias, Informed consent, Medical research, MSCs, Randomised Clinical trials, Sample size.

CHAPTER SUMMARY

Calculating the Appropriate Sample Size

- Use the MCID for sample size calculation, if there are no previous estimates in the literature.
- Increase the sample size by 20% to account for possible drop outs.
- To overcome low recruitment, multicenter clinical trial design is recommended.

Participant Selection

- Healthy volunteers should not be included in any phase of these trials.

---

* Corresponding author Ahmed S. Negida: Faculty of Medicine, Zagazig University, Zagazig, El-Sharkia, 44519 Egypt; Tel: +201125549087; E-mail: ahmed01251@medicine.zu.edu.eg

- Patients with established tissue degeneration should be included.
- All patients to be assessed at the baseline should be stratified according to the disease stage.

Informed Consent Pocess

- Clarify patients' misconceptions about stem cell interventions.
- Do not overestimate or underestimate the safety and efficacy of the intervention.

Avoiding the Expertise Bias

- Adopt the expertise based trial design where patients are allocated to experienced surgeons, first, and then allocated to the treatment groups.

Training Surgeons to Practice Novel Techniques

- A standard training should be provided to practicing surgeons who are involved in the clinical trial.

Outcome Measures

- Both radiological evidence and clinical measures should be considered in the clinical trial endpoints.

Blinding

- In case that blinding of the intervention is not feasible, the assessor blinded design should be adopted.

Handling Missing Data of Lost Patients

- Missing data should be handled by appropriate analysis according to the intention to treat principal.
- In case of ITT analysis based on the worst-case scenario, the best-case scenario should be assumed as well to avoid underestimating an intervention.

Clinical Trial Reporting

- Adhere to the CONSORT statement guidelines when reporting a clinical trial.
- Clinical trial results should be made publicly available within 24 months from completion of the trial (in compliance with the new WHO requirements).

Clinical Trial Data Sharing

- Whenever possible, the investigators should reidentified the patients' data with other researchers to maximize benefit from patients' data (in compliance with

ICMJEs recommendations).

1. INTRODUCTION TO CLINICAL TRIALS

In scientific research, the experimental research design is advocated over the observational research designs as it allows the researcher to control the risk assignment to the study groups. Similarly, in the clinical research, clinical trials is a better research design than observational designs. The first description of randomized controlled trial (RCT) was done by the British epidemiologist Austin Bradford Hill in the landmark study of Streptomycin for pulmonary tuberculosis [1].

In clinical trials, patients are exposed to the risk factor (intervention as drug or surgery) intentionally by the researchers in the context of the research study. While in the observational study designs, such interventions are given to the patients as part of the routine practice.

Observational research designs suffer from the risk of confounding bias. It is important to eliminate such confounders when evaluating the safety and efficacy of new treatment modalities. Clinical trials allow for minimizing the confounding bias by the randomization of patients to the treatment groups during the allocation process. Since randomization is the only scientific method that can adjust for known and unknown confounders, the resulting groups from this process will be nearly equal in all variables including known and unknown confounders (*i.e.* genetic factors). The only difference between the two randomized groups will be the provided treatment, therefore, at the end of the follow up period, any difference between these treatments should be attributed to the treatment and only to the treatment.

2. PHASES OF CLINICAL TRIALS

Clinical trials are classified into 4 phases:

Phase I Clinical Trials

• It aims at exploring the safety of the intervention on human population.
• Usually include small sample size (about 20-30 patients).
• No control group (usually, phase I clinical trials are single arm studies).
• The minimum dose of the intervention is given to avoid complications.

Phase II Clinical Trials

• They aim at proving the concept of drug efficacy.
• They include larger sample size than phase I studies (100-200 patients).

• Studies in this phase might be controlled by a placebo group.
• Complications and adverse events are recorded in this phase.

Phase III Clinical Trials

• They aim at proving the efficacy of the drug against other treatments.
• They include large sample size (300-1000 patients).
• These studies are large RCTs, the control group might be with a placebo group or another treatment or both.
• Various doses are explored in this phase and adverse events should be controlled in this phase of trials.

Phase IV Clinical Trials

They are postmarketing studies where data from consumers are collected and analyzed. Because some adverse events might require long induction period or might be of small but clinically significant effect size (ES), they do not occur when testing the intervention in the previous phases of clinical trials.

Stem Cell Trials in Orthopedic Surgery

The development of new therapies using stem cell in orthopedic patients is still challenging. Due to the novelty of these treatment strategies and the uncertainty about their safety and efficacy, clinical trials in this field require special ethical and methodological considerations.

Maintaining a Plausible Risk Benefit Ratio

Usually clinical trials involve both the potential benefits and risks to the participants. It is an ethical obligation that researchers do their best to minimize the potential risks and maximize the benefit to patients and to the scientific community. In the previous chapters, we have discussed the ethical challenges facing stem cell research in orthopedics, in this chapter, we are discussing the methodological principles that investigators should follow in orthopedic stem cell trials to ensure a proper design, high internal validity, attainable scientific knowledge, and to avoid potential bias during the study.

3. CALCULATING THE APPROPRIATE SAMPLE SIZE

Calculating the appropriate sample size is an important methodological issue in clinical trials. It is important that the sample size of the clinical study is sufficient to represent the effect size (ES). The statistical power is defined as the ability of the sample size to represent the ES. Most of clinical studies are designed with an 80% or 90% statistical power to detect the expected ES with an alpha level of 5%.

When calculating the sample size, the expected ES is assumed based on one of the following methods: (1) expert opinion, (2) pilot study by the investigators, (3) a previously published study, (4) minimum clinically important difference (MCID). (Table **1**).

Table 1. shows the methods of assuming the ES when calculating the sample size and the disadvantages and advantages of each method.

	Disadvantage	Advantage
Expert opinion	• The expert opinion might be biased to overestimate or underestimate the efficacy of the intervention.	• It is easy to obtain
Pilot study by the investigators	• The pilot study might not be feasible in stem cell orthopedic surgeries.	• Allow the researchers to calculate the sample size based on preliminary estimates derived from the same population of their clinical trial.
A previously published study	• In novel interventions, there may be no previous clinical studies about their efficacy. • Published studies might subject to variability due to difference in place, time, study population, used devices and systems.	• It might be easier for some researchers to rely on a similar previously published study.
MCID [2]	• The MCID might be too small and therefore, it will require a large sample size which is not practical in some cases.	• It does not require previous studies or an expert estimation. • Calculating the sample size based on this method (MCID) is always feasible.

Clinical trials in orthopedic surgery faces the risk of low recruitment for many reasons: Firstly, stem cell therapy is a novel strategy that has not approved yet for many orthopedic problems. Therefore, the number of patients interested in joining a clinical trial will be limited due to the usual fear of applying new procedures. Secondly, not all patients with orthopedic problems will be eligible to join these clinical trials owing to the ethical restrictions applied on participants' selection for stem cell trials that we have discussed previously.

Low recruitment of clinical trials can lead to a small sample size and therefore, the clinical trial will have an inadequate statistical power. It has been advocated that such clinical trials (underpowered clinical trials) are not ethical since they expose the patients to risks without generating the sufficient knowledge that the study was designed for.

In this regard, we recommend that:

1. Stem cell trials in orthopedic surgery should recruit patients from multiple centers. Such collaborative effort will help overcoming the problem of low

recruitment.
2. The appropriate sample size should be calculated to allow an 80% or 90% statistical power to detect the expected ES (usually, we consider the ES of the primary endpoint).
3. In case that the investigators cannot find any previous information to provide and approximate values for the efficacy of this intervention, we recommend that the ES used for sample size calculation will be the MCID.

Example for Sample Size Calculation

We are designing a parallel RCT to investigate the efficacy of postoperative platelet-rich plasma injections on arthroscopic supraspinatus repair in terms of constant strength score after 4 years.

Therefore, we hypothesize the following regarding the constant strength score

H1: PRP group > control group (*mean difference >0*)

H0: PRP group = control group *or* PRP group < control group (*mean difference ≤0*)

A literature search of PubMed (last accessed 1st, February 2018) showed that Ebert *et al*. [3] was the most recent relevant study reporting the efficacy of this intervention. The study of Ebert *et al*. reported a mean difference between the two groups of 3.3 points with 95% CI (1.0 to 5.7), and the standard deviation of the constant strength scores were 6.3 and 6.6 for the PRP and control groups, respectively.

Therefore,

• The ES is represented as the mean difference between the PRP and the control groups from the baseline to endpoint. The expected mean difference in our new study will be assumed to be 3.3 points
• The population standard deviation is about 6.5 points.

To detect this ES with a 90% power and a 5% probability of type I error under a two-sided hypothesis, a minimum sample size of 166 patients is required (n=83 per group assuming a 1:1 allocation ratio).

These calculations were done on *SampSize app* (for android version 8.0.0 [www]). The detailed steps of the calculation are illustrated on Figs. (**1-3**).

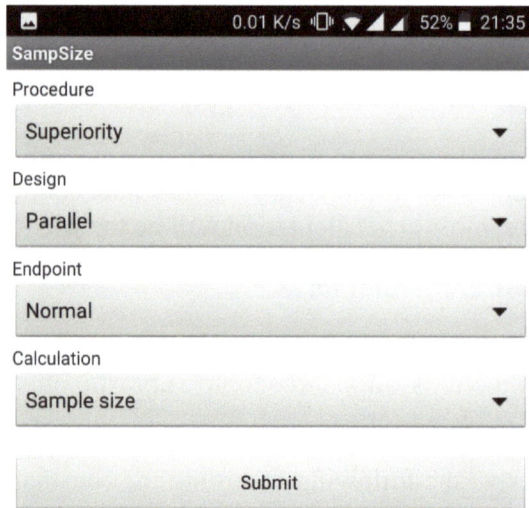

Fig. (1). Shows sample size calculation steps on SampSize app for android (First step: selecting the type of the clinical trial design and the type of endpoint).

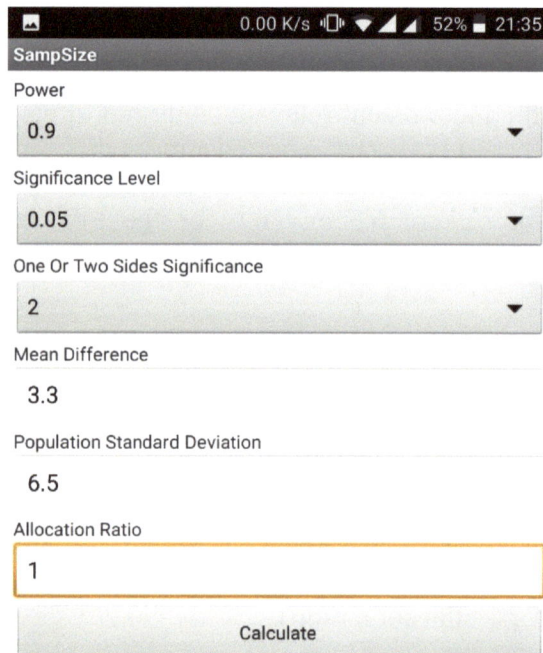

Fig. (2). Shows sample size calculation steps on SampSize app for android. (Second step: selecting the study power and significance level and submitting the expected mean difference between the two groups and the population SD).

```
📷                    0.03 K/s  ◐ ▼ ◢ ◢ 52% ■ 21:35
Results
```

Power
0.90

Significance Level
0.050

One Or Two Sided Significance
2

Mean Difference
3.300

Population Standard Deviation
6.500

Allocation Ratio
1.000

Sample Size Group 1
83

Sample Size Group 2
83

Total Sample Size
166

References

Julious, SA. Sample sizes for clinical trials. Chapman and Hall, 2009

Julious, S. A. (2004). Tutorial in Biostatistics:Sample sizes for clinical trials with Normal Data. Statistics in Medicine, 23, 1921-86

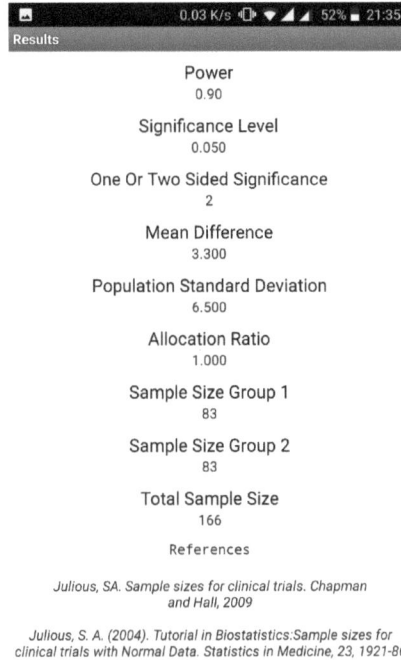

Fig. (3). Shows sample size calculation steps on SampSize app for android (The study will require a minimum sample size of 166 patients).

4. PARTICIPANT SELECTION

Selecting appropriate participants for stem cell clinical trials in orthopedics is challenging. As we explained previously that the variations among patients in disease stage and the level of disability will account in a different microenvironment and therefore, might cause a difference in the mechanism of action, magnitude of improvement, and the potential risks and complications of the intervention.

The health status of individuals is an important determinant for selecting patients to such trials. Regenerative medicine field is interested in making interventions for early-stage disease to prevent the need for symptomatic strategies introducing the intervention into viable microenvironment. However, in some conditions, it might be difficult to identify early-stage patients as many patients are undiagnosed at the early disease stage and it will be difficult to define and detect a significant tissue degeneration to justify the need for interventions. Nevertheless, stable enrolling early-stage subjects are not favorable in the case of stem cell therapy due to the risk of having an unnecessary treatment, receiving a potentially unsafe intervention that might affect their functionality. On the other hand, stable patients eligible for conducting early clinical studies are at high risk of developing degeneration [4].

Patients with a late-stage disease are those terminally ill patients who are appropriate to assess the safety and potential efficacy of stem cell in orthopedic RCTs, because these patients cannot lose much more functionality, unless the consequences of the intervention affect the surrounding and remaining tissue [5]. On the other hand, the potential benefits for these patients may be lower due to the less suitable microenvironment for the stem cells [4].

Given that phase I trials aim at assessing the general safety of the intervention in the study population in a single arm design, enrolling healthy volunteers to this phase of stem cell trials is unethical, instead, patients with terminal stage of the disease are better selected for such trials since they do not have so much to lose. In the subsequent phases of clinical trials (phase II and phase III), the study population should be patients with stable disease with evidence of a significant tissue degeneration. Patients in this phase of trials should be stratified according to the stage of the disease and the severity of symptoms. The assessment of the disease stage based on radiological findings and the severity of patient symptoms should be done at the baseline evaluation (day 0 of the trial).

In summary, participant selection should subject to the following recommendations:

- Healthy volunteers should *not* be enrolled in any phase of these trials
- Only patients with significant tissue degeneration are eligible
- Expertise based trial design should be performed; patients are allocated to the experienced surgeons first, then allocated to the treatment groups
- The disease stage should be assessed at the baseline and patients to be stratified according to disease stage in the final analysis

5. THE INFORMED CONSENT PROCESS

In clinical studies where investigators are in direct communication with the study personnel, obtaining an informed consent is obligatory as per ethics principals.

In the informed consent process, investigators inform the participants about the study methodology, purpose, risks and benefits. Investigators should explain to the participants how the intervention might work and the expected risks and benefits based on previous studies. Then, patients make their decision about whether they agree to enroll in this study. A written informed consent is given as a guarantee that the patients were informed about the study details and agree voluntarily to participate in the study. In developing countries where some of the study population might be illiterate, a detailed and simplified explanation of the study details should be provided and an oral informed consent in the presence of a third party, can be obtained. In case of the participant cannot give this consent due to any disability, an alternative preventative should write this informed consent instead of the patient himself.

It is important here to mention that patients might have misconceptions about stem cell therapy. Stem cell interventions have recently gained a lot of interest and many companies endorse these products in their propaganda and tend to overestimate the potential of stem cell interventions. In addition, orthopedic surgeons themselves might be too optimistic and overestimate or underestimate the safety and efficacy of stem cell interventions. Therefore, in stem cell trials, orthopedic surgeons should be conscious about the information they provide to the patients and should also avoid any overestimation or underestimation. It is their duty to provide those subjects with accurate information about the surgery such as procedures, nature, and duration of the clinical trial, alternative solution as other types of surgery, or even treatment if available, and finally allow them to freely discuss their inquiries regarding the surgery in order to correct their believes and misconceptions. This information should be clarified completely to the potential participants prior to enrolling in the clinical trial. After that, the participants should sign a written informed consent.

Moreover, all the participants should have the right to leave the study at any point without losing of the benefits to which they are otherwise entitled. Clinicians should follow up their patients after transplantation to ensure their safety.

6. THE EXPERTISE-BASED TRIAL DESIGN

Expertise Bias is a critical point when conducting orthopedic surgery RCTs. For example, to run a clinical trial of bone regeneration, we should have qualified and motivated surgeons to ensure the safety and wellbeing of the study participants. Generally, in the new surgical techniques, there are variations in surgeons' skills and their ability to perform a new strategy in his surgery. This problem is best solved, as discussed previously [6], by designing the "expertise-based clinical trial" [7] in which the allocation of the study subjects is done based on the treatment provider not to the treatment itself in order to ensure the expertise and motivation of the performing surgeons to avoid potential bias.

7. STANDARD TRAINING OF THE INVOLVED SURGEONS

Nevertheless, stem cell therapy RCTs will face the problem that such treatment modalities have not been approved, yet. As a result, most orthopedic surgeons do not have prior experience in stem cell injection and handling. This problem could be overcome by providing a standard training to the orthopedic surgeons involved in the RCTs. This training includes an explanation of the surgical approaches used during the introduction of the stem cells. The training also is important to ensure a standardized implementation of the intervention.

8. COMBINING RADIOLOGICAL AND CLINICAL OUTCOME MEASURES

In orthopedic surgeries, both clinical symptoms and radiological evidence are important when determining the efficacy of an intervention. As we mentioned previously that radiography might show evidence of bone healing while the patient still suffers from pain or disability. Therefore, we recommend that in stem cell trials, investigators should combine radiological evidence with clinical assessment in the primary and secondary endpoints.

9. PATIENT ASSESSMENT USING THE ASSESSOR BLINDED DESIGN

In clinical trials, blinding is done to ensure that patients (and sometimes the physicians) are not aware about the intervention to-which the patients are allocated and therefore minimize the risk of performance bias in the trial. However, in many surgeries including orthopedic interventions, blinding is not possible. Additionally, we mentioned earlier that using a sham surgery or a placebo intervention might not be ethical in such surgical interventions leaving the trial with open label design where the patients and surgeons are fully aware about the intervention allocated to the study participants. We recommend that the assessor blinded trial design might help to minimize such risk of bias. The assessor blinded design means that patient assessment, at the evaluation points of a clinical trial, is done by blinded clinicians who are not aware about the intervention allocated to those patients.

10. HANDLING MISSING DATA WITH APPROPRIATE ANALYSIS

Loss of patients during the follow up is not uncommon in clinical trials. The differential loss of patients between the two study groups might result in attrition bias. As a result, the clinical trial design will suffer from two problems.

The first problem (decreasing the study power): Losing patients from the clinical trial will reduce the final sample size which affects the statistical power of the study and might leave the study *underpowered.*

Solution: To overcome the first problem, many investigators increase the sample size of the study by the expected dropout rate. Therefore, investigators should take into consideration the expected drop-out rate from their study and add this rate to the calculated sample size (+20% is commonly used for such calculation).

Therefore, losing some patients from the study is not likely to threaten the study power after drop outs as we have planned for these drop-outs from the beginning.

The second problem (misbalancing confounders): In RCTs, the differential loss of patients from the study groups will misbalance the random distribution of confounders between the two groups *threatening the internal validity* of the RCT.

Solution: It is worth notice that increasing the sample size before the study will fix the first problem (study power) but will not solve the second problem (misbalancing confounders) even if the study power remained high after drop-outs. To understand this problem, we should consider the following points:

- Randomization is the only scientific method that can ensure balancing known and unknown confounders between the study groups, therefore, any differences between these two groups after the follow up will be attributed to the intervention only.
- This key element (randomization) makes RCTs of high internal validity and allows to eliminate confounders and explore the treatment efficacy in a pragmatic approach within the clinical trial environment.
- The presence of each patient in his study group is important to maintain balance between confounders, therefore, losing some patients from the study will misbalance these confounders and threaten the internal validity. Even adding more patients to the study will not fix this misbalance because investigators are not aware which confounders are implicated given that randomization account for unknown confounders as well (for example: genetic factors).

Because the presence of each patient in his study group is important to maintain balance between confounders, all randomized patients should be included in the final analysis irrespective to any withdrawals from the study groups. Therefore, the term *"intention to treat"* principal was introduced. In the ITT analysis, all randomized patients are considered for the final analysis irrespective of any withdrawals. Another question arises here: How can we obtain the endpoint values of lost patients?

(1) From hospital records and death certificates

If the hospital is part of the health system network in your area, you can know whether the patient is seeking medical treatment elsewhere. If the patient dies, you can identify this from the death certificates record in your area.

(2) Last observation carried forward analysis (LOCF analysis)

In this model, we assume that the last observation of each lost patient is their endpoint. For example, in a clinical trial extending for 12 months, patients were followed up regularly every 3 months. If some patients were lost from the final visit, the LOCF analysis assumes that the 9th month visit is the endpoint of the lost patients.

(3) Multiple imputations

This is a statistical method where we use patient values during the regular visits to predict the endpoint values of the final visit. This statistical method is based on regression models and adding some random numbers to calculate the predicted endpoint values of lost patients.

(4) Analysis of the worst-case scenario

In this model, we assume the worst scenario for all lost patients from the study groups. The worst case is defined as the participant with the best baseline and worst endpoint of the completed patients. The endpoint values of the worst case are assigned to lost patients, while their original demographic characteristics and their prior visit values are still considered for the analysis.

(5) Analysis of the best-case scenario

The scenario of the worst case has been criticized by pharmaceutical industry and some methodologists because it might underestimate the treatment efficacy in both groups. To balance the worst-case scenario, the best-case scenario was introduced where we assigned values of the best patient to the lost cases. However, this might overestimate the treatment efficacy if done alone. Therefore, both scenarios are recommended to be done together.

We recommend that in an RCT where lost patient data could not be obtained for analysis, the investigators should analyze their data based on the ITT principal in the worst-case and best-case scenarios. If the treatment was found superior in both analysis scenarios, we will be confident of its superiority whatever the values of lost patients were.

11. CLINICAL TRIAL REPORTING

Recently, standard reporting of clinical studies has been endorsed with the development of EQUATOR network [www], where clinical research scientists are developing standard reporting checklists to ensure investigators are reporting sufficient details about their studies in the final publications. Many of the top-tier journals nowadays ask the investigators to submit the standard reporting checklist align with their manuscript to act as an index for their research papers and ensure that all elements of the clinical study are reported. For clinical trials, the

CONSORT statement[www] has been developed and is widely endorser by medical journals, pharmaceuticals, and funding agencies.

It should not escape our notice that publishing clinical trial results is now obligatory for all registered studies. In April 2015, the WHO issued the public disclosure of clinical trial results statement [www] which implies that *"(1) the main findings of clinical trials are to be submitted for publication in a peer reviewed journal within 12 months of study completion and are to be published through an open access mechanism unless there is a specific reason why open access cannot be used, or otherwise made available publicly at most within 24 months of study completion, and (2) In addition, the key outcomes are to be made publicly available within 12 months of study completion by posting to the results section of the primary clinical trial registry. Where a registry is used without a results database available, the results should be posted on a free-to-access, publicly available, searchable institutional website of the Regulatory Sponsor, Funder or Principal Investigator"*. This statement prevents the control of pharmaceuticals and funding agencies who sometimes withhold the publication of clinical trial results if the results do not seem favorable from their point of view. Since patients exposed themselves to risks and agreed to participate in the study, it is a moral obligation to publish these results to the scientific community.

12. CLINICAL TRIAL DATA SHARING

Villain and colleagues investigated the feasibility of obtaining individual patient data from orthopedic surgery RCTs [8]. They identified 38 research questions and 273 relevant RCTs. They emailed the 273 corresponding authors, however, they got only 37 positive response. This study highlights the problem of data sharing especially in orthopedic surgery. In January 2016, the international committee of medical journal editors (ICMJEs) issued a proposal for data sharing statement, and the final statement was issued in June 2017 [www] confirming that editors will take into consideration data sharing statements when making editorial decisions. Many ICMJEs member journals will mandate and adopt specific requirements for data sharing of clinical trials. This step is crucial to maximize the benefit from patient data and fulfilling the moral obligation towards research participants who put themselves at risk during the clinical trial. In stem cell trials, the low recruitment due to fears of a new intervention and the expertise-based allocation will make the study population more vulnerable and will obligate more need to maximize the benefit from their data through data sharing and collaboration with other research groups and institutions to push the process forward.

WEBSITES

• SampSize app: https://www.epigenesys.org.uk/portfolio/sampsize/

- Equator network: http://www.equator-network.org/
- CONSORT statement: http://www.consort-statement.org/
- WHO statement of public disclosure of clinical trials: http://www.who.int/ entity/ictrp/results/WHO_Statement_results_reporting_clinical_trials.pdf?ua=1
- ICMJEs' data sharing statement: http://icmje.org/news-and-editorials/data_ sharing_june_2017.pdf

CONSENT FOR PUBLICATION

Not applicable.

CONFLICT OF INTEREST

The authors declare no conflict of interest, financial or otherwise.

ACKNOWLEDGEMENTS

Declared none.

REFERENCES

[1]   A Medical Research Council Investigation. STREPTOMYCIN treatment of pulmonary tuberculosis. Br Med J 1948; 2: 769-82.

[2]   Bernstein J, Mcguire K. Part II. Statistical issues in the design of orthopaedic studies statistical sampling and hypothesis testing in orthopaedic research. 2003; 55–62.

[3]   Ebert JR, Wang A, Smith A, *et al.* A Midterm Evaluation of Postoperative Platelet-Rich Plasma Injections on Arthroscopic Supraspinatus Repair: A Randomized Controlled Trial. Am J Sports Med 2017; 45(13): 2965-74.
        [http://dx.doi.org/10.1177/0363546517719048] [PMID: 28806095]

[4]   Niemansburg SL, van Delden JJ, Dhert WJ, Bredenoord AL. Regenerative medicine interventions for orthopedic disorders: ethical issues in the translation into patients. Regen Med 2013; 8(1): 65-73.
        [http://dx.doi.org/10.2217/rme.12.112] [PMID: 23259806]

[5]   Niemansburg SL, Delden JJM, Van , Dhert WJA, Bredenoord AL. Ethical implications of regenerative medicine in orthopedics : an empirical study with surgeons and scientists in the field 2013

[6]   Poolman RW, Hanson B, Marti RK, Bhandari M. Conducting a clinical study: A guide for good research practice. Indian J Orthop 2007; 41(1): 27-31.
        [http://dx.doi.org/10.4103/0019-5413.30522] [PMID: 21124679]

[7]   Devereaux PJ, Bhandari M, Clarke M, *et al.* Need for expertise based randomised controlled trials. BMJ 2005; 330(7482): 88.
        [http://dx.doi.org/10.1136/bmj.330.7482.88] [PMID: 15637373]

[8]   Villain B, Dechartres A, Boyer P, Ravaud P. Feasibility of individual patient data meta-analyses in orthopaedic surgery. BMC Med 2015; 13: 131.
        [http://dx.doi.org/10.1186/s12916-015-0376-6] [PMID: 26040278]

Bone Marrow Aspirate Concentrate, 2018, 51-59

CHAPTER 5

Role in Non-union and Bone Defects

Khaled Emara*, Ramy Ahmed Diab and **Ahmed K. Emara**

Orthopaedic surgery department, Ain Shams University, Cairo, Egypt

Abstract: Non-unions occur mostly due to fracture stability, decrease in blood supply, or both. The cause of non-union is subcategorised into biological and mechanical factors. There are several risk factors for non-union which include -but are not limited to smoking, diabetes mellitus, infection, open or compound fractures, senility, inadequate nutrition and some drugs like NSAIDs.

Mechanical factors include the application of electric fields, physical stimulation and ultrasound. The biological materials include osteoconductive agents such as tricalcium phosphate (TCP), hydroxyapatite (HA) preferably with added Osteoinductive agents, which enhance migration, proliferation and differentiation of cells to promote fracture healing. Such agents as Platelets rich plasma (PRP), Bone marrow aspirate concentrate (BMAC), and Bone morphogenetic protein (BMP).

Keywords: Bone defects, Bone Marrow Aspirate Concentrate (BMAC), Delayed union, Expanded stem cells, Fracture, Malunion, MSCs, Non-union.

INTRODUCTION

Non-unions occur mostly due to fracture instability, vascular supply, or both. There are other several risk factors for non-union which include-but are not limited to smoking, diabetes mellitus, infection, open or compound fractures, senility, inadequate nutrition and some drugs like Non-steroidals.

Fracture healing involves a dynamic sequence, which eventually retains the functional and biomechanical bone integrity [1]. It is estimated that non-union may complicate 4.8 to 10% of fractures with the incidence varying according to fracture type and location.

Segmental bone graft transplant has been and still is the golden choice for treating osseous defects and non-unions. However, an increasing number of papers are challenging this notion and placing several alternatives that can replace bone

---
* **Corresponding author Khaled Emara:** Orthopaedic surgery department, Ain Shams University, Cairo, Egypt; Tel: +20222055661; Fax: +20222055662; E-mail: Kmemara@hotmail.com

grafting or say the least, be used in combination with it to produce superior results. These newer alternatives vary widely representing both physical as well as biological agents.

Mechanical factors include the application of electric fields, physical stimulation and ultrasound. The biological materials include osteoconductive agents such as tricalcium phosphate (TCP), hydroxyapatite (HA) preferably with added osteoinductive agents which enhance migration, proliferation and differentiation of cells to promote fracture healing. Such agents as Platelets rich plasma (PRP), Bone marrow aspirate concentrate (BMAC), and Bone morphogenetic protein (BMP).

Therefore, the idea is to use osteoinductive material (such as BMAC) in an osteoconductive matrix to drive the regeneration of bone [2]. There is progressively increasing interest in the use of BMAC as an osteoinductive material for bone regeneration [3].

Bone marrow aspirate concentrate (BMAC) was first described in 1952 in the context of being an extension of the already in use iliac crest bone graft [4]. A previous practice was to expand the small number of mesenchymal stem cells obtained by aspiration, then subject the patient to another procedure to inject the in-vitro propagated cell lines, which become available in greater numbers than when aspirated and thus, greater concentrations. This previous practice is of significance in the treatment of chondral lesions. However, this practice has been replaced by the concentration of the bone marrow aspirate then reinjecting in one step, which serves the purpose of increasing the number of progenitor cells and a number of growth factors per millilitre thereby, delivering an increased concentration of osteoinductive material within the same operation. This avoids the need for *in vitro* propagation of the aspirated progenitor cells with its increased costs and risk of complications such as infection as well as the complications associated with most two-step surgeries [4].

One of the earliest studies undertaken on the applications of BMAC was conducted by Hernigou *et al.* who advocated that the released growth factors from the bone marrow are effective in the fracture healing [5]. Goujon *et al.* used rabbits to demonstrate the osteogenic effects of BMAC [6]. Ever since then many studies have discussed the possible clinical applications of BMAC in orthopaedic surgery and the efficacy of its use. The earliest encouraging results from BMAC were demonstrated by Jäger *et al.*, who emphasized the safety of harvesting, concentration, and stimulation of osteogenic differentiation by BMAC injection in the transplant site without requiring further external stimuli to promote this differentiation [7].

THE COMBINED USE OF BMAC AND PRP

The addition of PRP to BMAC has been proven to increase the bone regenerative effects of BMACs mononuclear cells. The mechanism of action of the added PRP is mainly *via* growth factor release from the platelet alpha granules. These growth factors and cytokines act upon the MSCs leading to their proliferation and differentiation into osteoblasts. In addition to their osteoinductive effect the growth factors also stimulate angiogenesis [10]. Dong Hoon Lee *et al.* emphasized the significance of using a combination of BMAC and PRP in distraction osteogenesis in patients undergoing bilateral tibial lengthening. Results indicated that patients receiving this combination had improved bone healing during distraction with better anterior, posterior, medial and lateral cortical healing indices as well as earlier weight bearing than patients who did not receive this combination. However, the external fixation index as well as the size and shape of the callus showed no significant difference between both groups of patients. It was also postulated that the use of the combination of BMAC and PRP would be more effective if injected during the distraction phase rather than at the end of a distraction given that immunohistochemical analyses shown great expression of growth receptors in distraction period [11]. In another study performed on 32 minipigs, the radiological and histomorphological analysis demonstrated significantly higher bone formation in an osseous defect in the group treated with BMAC plus PRP on a calcium phosphate glass scaffold compared to BMAC on CPG scaffold [12]. The nature and the mechanism of action of this combination treatment still require verification by future studies [11]. It still remains unclear whether the favourable outcomes of BMAC/PRP combination are a result of a single component with one element having the upper hand in the regenerative effect or is it a synergistic effect between a numbers of elements [13].

SCAFFOLDS

One of the determinants of BMAC effectiveness in bone regeneration is the scaffold used for implantation. Collagen-sponge scaffolds provide good cell adherence *in vitro*; however, they are quickly resorbed *in vivo* and therefore lack the biomechanical support needed to achieve early weight bearing [14]. Moreover, this rapid degradation of the collagen-sponge scaffold *in vivo* diminishes its cell-guiding function observed *in vitro* [15]. In addition to its rapid dissolution, the scaffold is of a viscoelastic nature making it very difficult to fill bone defects with a complex geometry [10]. One study has compared the use of collagen-sponge scaffolds *versus* Hydroxyapatite crystals in terms of the time to bone healing, early weight bearing and cell attachment for each of the two scaffold types. Results showed that despite the Hydroxyapatite scaffolds having less cell adhesion *in vitro* than the collagen-sponge scaffolds, they actually achieve faster bone regeneration as well as earlier weight bearing This is in part owing to its delayed resorption *in vivo* compared to the collagen-sponge scaffold, thereby allowing more structural support). These characteristics of hydroxyapatite scaffolds have made their use more favourable especially in weight-bearing areas where the risk of refracture is high and the rapidly resorbed collagen-sponge scaffold with its lack of biomechanical functions will not be able to provide adequately prolonged support. It is thought that collagen hydroxyapatite scaffolds could, in fact, achieve the benefits of both types [7].

INDICATIONS

The earliest studies on the indications for use of BMAC were tibial shaft fractures due to their high rates of nonunion [16]. Subsequently, BMAC has been integrated into studies of different lesions requiring enhancement of the cellular proliferation and healing [17]. This interest was not limited to BMAC application in the treatment of non-unions but extended to all types of osseous defects as well as distraction osteogenesis [18]. BMAC has also been used successfully in treatment of talus and knee osteochondritis desiccants lesions.

It has also been used to assist in the integration of osteochondral allograft plugs. BMAC use has been reported in different types of fractures with the common indication being the need for enhanced healing at the site of use [4]. An important advantage of BMAC that must be taken into consideration is that it is a type of auto-transplant, which decreases the chances of associated disease transmission as well as obliterating any possibility of immunogenic reactions. Both complications, on the other hand, are present with the utilization of synthetic and allogenic material [19].

DISTRACTION OSTEOGENESIS OF THE TIBIA

Distraction osteogenesis is recognized as an essential method in reconstructive surgery.

Enhancing bone formation, avoiding complications as bone non-union or mal-union as well as facilitating early fixator removal. Also it permits early weight bearing and the early back to life activities [11]. Many factors influence bone regeneration have been demonstrated [20]: (1) Host factors, such as age, segment defect, and systemic disease (2) Local causes, as poor soft tissue status and infection (3) Surgeon factors, as inadequate soft tissue handling, poor osteotomy type and technique selection, unstable fixation method, and improper distraction rate and rhythm.

Dong Hoon Lee *et al.* emphasized the significance of using a combination of BMAC and PRP in distraction osteogenesis in cases with bilateral tibial lengthening. The BMAC+PRP combination had improved healing in distraction with better anterior, posterior, medial and lateral cortical healing indices as well as earlier weight bearing than patients who did not receive this combination. However, the external fixation index, as well as the size and shape of the callus demonstrated no significant difference between both groups. It is suggested that the use of the combination of BMAC and PRP is more effective when injected during the distraction phase rather than after the end of distraction.

The scaffold provided by the natural fibrovascular lattice created between the two distracted bone ends during the distraction process, acting as a membranous tube in which BMAC can be injected and suspended [8]. Immunohistochemical analyses indirectly support the administration of BMAC during the distraction phase, since it was shown that great expression of growth receptors in distraction period However, this still requires verification by future studies [11].

OSSEOUS DEFECTS (POTENTIAL OR ESTABLISHED NON-UNIONS)

Segmental defects can be created posttraumatic with bone loss, after resection of a tumour, osteolysis, pseudarthrosis and infections. Ever since the initiation of bone graft transfer and up till now, the bone graft has been the gold standard in smaller defects, up to 3 cm because cancellous bone grafts provide the essential requirements for bone regeneration, cells, bone-inductive proteins. Major complications of this method are donor-site morbidity, which may lead to pain, hematoma, or infection as well as being in itself a limited resource and one with decreased healing potential with aging [21]. In osseous defects over 3cm, the use of segmental bone transport remains the gold standard despite being long time consumption and associated complications as infection, pseudoarthrosis, etc. However, Petri *et al.* have shown that BMAC could be a viable as an alternative to bone transfer techniques for bone defects between 3cm and 7cm given the presence of a well-vascularized transplant site. For poorly vascularized transplant sites or bone defects over 7cm the use of BMAC to replace segmental bone transfer has not shown favourable results.

In another study, Gessmann *et al.* examined the percutaneous BMAC injection into the regenerated bone section in tibial bone defects that underwent Ilizarov segmental transport. They showed excellent bone healing and no complications in all patients [22]. A third study concluded that treating large long bone defects with stem cell concentrates can achieve good results, with early weight bearing [8]. Therefore, BMAC has the potential to overcome many of the limitations imposed by bone autografts in the treatment of osseous defects such as, the decrease of bone healing capability in old age, diseases with high recurrence including but not limited to aneurysmal bone cysts and congenital pseudarthrosis [23, 24]. Osteoporotic patients could also benefit from the use of BMAC as a part of their treatment in the presence of osseous defects [25]. This makes volumetric bone deficiencies which fit the previous criteria a solid indication for the use of BMAC. With this being said, further studies are required for the purpose of comparing the outcomes of using; BMAC alone, BMAC on scaffolds (collagen and hydroxyapatite), and BMAC with concurrent autologous segmental transfer *versus* the use of autologous segmental transfer alone [7, 10, 13]. It is also important to note that in a separate study BMAC was used in conjunction with TCP for treating osseous defects with no reported benefits. These statements serve to clarify the still on-going controversy on the extent of the benefit provided by BMAC and the need for further studies in this field [4].

Distraction osteogenesis is well known procedure treating segmental bone defects. But has the disadvantages of the long duration in bulky external fixator with patients' discomfort. Currently, application of percutaneous adjuvants to reduce time one consolidation is one of the major goals in the up-coming research. Kitoh *et al.* demonstrated that percutaneous platelet-rich and plasma transplantation of culture-expanded bone marrow cells enhances bone regeneration during distraction osteogenesis [26]. However, there are still some risks, as contamination or depletion of proliferative capacity, as well as high costs [10].

Hernigou *et al.* showed that efficacy seems to be related to the number of progenitor cells in the graft [27]. A reported indication of implementing BMAC treatment is bone cysts even though repeated injections may be necessary [10]. Another indication for the use of BMAC (preferably in combination with PRP) is to achieve spinal fusion, especially in multi-level operations in patients predisposed to pseudo-arthrosis and in elderly multi-diseased osteoporotic patients [10, 28]. This will be explained in details later in this book.

BONES FRACTURE OF THE FIFTH METATARSAL

The use of BMAC in the treatment of fifth metatarsal bones fracture has been shown to be beneficial when added to the routinely used internal fixation. This could be attributed to the compromised vascularity of this watershed area where the blood supply *via* the nutrient artery is interrupted by the fracture pattern. BMAC, in this case, helped to promote the biological activity, which along with the stability of internal fixation was an adequate solution to the non-union, which can pose a considerable challenge, imposed especially in athletes [29].

OSTEOMYELITIS

The immunomodulatory properties of MSCs have the potential to prevent or treat infection. Hernigou *et al.* reported that local application of concentrated CFU GM derived colonies actually resolved infection and resulted in bone healing in an infected non-union of polytrauma patients. Although the technique of preparation of the aspirate is entirely different in this case, the study itself proves the versatility of the application of stem cell therapy in combating infections, especially with the increasing emergence of antibiotic-resistant strains. However, this application requires further studies [30].

CONSENT FOR PUBLICATION

Not applicable.

CONFLICT OF INTEREST

The authors declare no conflict of interest, financial or otherwise.

ACKNOWLEDGEMENTS

Declared none.

REFERENCES

[1]   Hannouche D, Petite H, Sedel L. Current trends in the enhancement of fracture healing. J Bone Joint Surg Br 2001; 83(2): 157-64.
[http://dx.doi.org/10.1302/0301-620X.83B2.12106] [PMID: 11284556]

[2]   Hierholzer C, Sama D, Toro JB, Peterson M, Helfet DL. Plate fixation of ununited humeral shaft fractures: effect of type of bone graft on healing. J Bone Joint Surg Am 2006; 88(7): 1442-7.
[PMID: 16818968]

[3]   Connolly JF, Guse R, Tiedeman J, Dehne R. Autologous marrow injection as a substitute for operative grafting of tibial nonunions 1991.
[http://dx.doi.org/10.1097/00003086-199105000-00038]

[4]   Smith B, Goldstein T, Ekstein C. Biologic adjuvants and bone: current use in orthopedic surgery. Curr Rev Musculoskelet Med 2015; 8(2): 193-9.
[http://dx.doi.org/10.1007/s12178-015-9265-z] [PMID: 25804684]

[5]   Hernigou P. Growth factors released from bone marrow are promising tools in orthopedic surgery. Rev Rhum Engl Ed 1998; 65(2): 79-84.
[PMID: 9540115]

[6]   Hernigou P, Poignard A, Manicom O, Mathieu G, Rouard H. The use of percutaneous autologous bone marrow transplantation in nonunion and avascular necrosis of bone. J Bone Joint Surg Br 2005; 87(7): 896-902.
[http://dx.doi.org/10.1302/0301-620X.87B7.16289] [PMID: 15972899]

[7]   Jager M, Herten M, Fochtmann U. Bridging the gap: bone marrow aspiration concentrate reduces autologous bone grafting in osseous defects 2011; J Orthop Res 29(2):173–180.

[8]   Petri M, Namazian A, Wilke F, *et al.* Repair of segmental long-bone defects by stem cell concentrate

augmented scaffolds: a clinical and positron emission tomography--computed tomography analysis. Int Orthop 2013; 37(11): 2231-7.
[http://dx.doi.org/10.1007/s00264-013-2087-y] [PMID: 24013459]

[9]   Torres J, Lopes A, Lopes MA, Gutierres A, Cabral AT, Fernandes MH, *et al.* The benefit of a human bone marrow stem cells concentrate in addition to an inorganic scaffold for bone regeneration: an *in vitro* study. Biomed Res Int 2015; 2015: 240698 Published online 2015 Jan 22.

[10]   Jäger M, Jelinek EM, Wess KM, *et al.* Bone marrow concentrate: a novel strategy for bone defect treatment. Curr Stem Cell Res Ther 2009; 4(1): 34-43.
[http://dx.doi.org/10.2174/157488809787169039] [PMID: 19149628]

[11]   Lee DH, Ryu KJ, Kim JW, Kang KC, Choi YR. Bone marrow aspirate concentrate and platelet-rich plasma enhanced bone healing in distraction osteogenesis of the tibia. Clin Orthop Relat Res 2014.
[http://dx.doi.org/10.1007/s11999-014-3548-]

[12]   Hakimi M, Grassmann JP, Betsch M, *et al.* The composite of bone marrow concentrate and PRP as an alternative to autologous bone grafting. PLoS One 2014; 9(6): e100143.
[http://dx.doi.org/10.1371/journal.pone.0100143] [PMID: 24950251]

[13]   Petri M, Namazian A, Wilke F, *et al.* Repair of segmental long-bone defects by stem cell concentrate augmented scaffolds: a clinical and positron emission tomography--computed tomography analysis. Int Orthop 2013; 37(11): 2231-7. [SICOT].
[http://dx.doi.org/10.1007/s00264-013-2087-y] [PMID: 24013459]

[14]   Knutsen G, Engebretsen L, Ludvigsen TC, *et al.* Autologous chondrocyte implantation compared with microfracture in the knee. A randomized trial. J Bone Joint Surg Am 2004; 86-A(3): 455-64.
[http://dx.doi.org/10.2106/00004623-200403000-00001] [PMID: 14996869]

[15]   Marx RE, Tursun R. A qualitative and quantitative analysis of autologous human multipotent adult stem cells derived from three anatomic areas by marrow aspiration: tibia, anterior ilium, and posterior ilium 2013.
[http://dx.doi.org/10.11607/jomi.te10]

[16]   Arbeloa-Gutierrez L, Dean CS, Chahla J, Pascual-Garrido C. Core decompression augmented with autologous bone marrow aspiration concentrate for early avascular necrosis of the femoral head. Arthrosc Tech 2016; 5(3): e615-20.
[http://dx.doi.org/10.1016/j.eats.2016.02.009] [PMID: 27656386]

[17]   Vulcano E, Murena L, Falvo DA, Baj A, Toniolo A, Cherubino P. Bone marrow aspirate and bone allograft to treat acetabular bone defects in revision total hip arthroplasty: preliminary report. Eur Rev Med Pharmacol Sci 2013; 17(16): 2240-9.
[PMID: 23893192]

[18]   de Oliveira TA, Aloise AC, Orosz JE, *et al.* Double centrifugation *versus* single centrifugation of bone marrow Aspirate concentrate in sinus floor elevation: a pilot study. Int J Oral Maxillofac Implants 2016; 31(1): 216-22.
[http://dx.doi.org/10.11607/jomi.4170] [PMID: 26800181]

[19]   Flouzat-Lachaniette CH, Heyberger C, Bouthors C, *et al.* Osteogenic progenitors in bone marrow aspirates have clinical potential for tibial non-unions healing in diabetic patients. Int Orthop 2016; 40(7): 1375-9.
[http://dx.doi.org/10.1007/s00264-015-3046-6] [PMID: 26572889]

[20]   Burkhart KJ, Rommens PM. Intramedullary application of bone morphogenetic protein in the management of a major bone defect after an Ilizarov procedure. J Bone Joint Surg Br 2008; 90(6): 806-9.
[http://dx.doi.org/10.1302/0301-620X.90B6.20147] [PMID: 18539677]

[21]   Meister K, Segal D, Whitelaw GP. The role of bone grafting in the treatment of delayed unions and nonunions of the tibia. Orthop Rev 1990; 19(3): 260-71.
[PMID: 2184392]

[22] Gessmann J, Köller M, Godry H, Schildhauer TA, Seybold D. Regenerate augmentation with bone marrow concentrate after traumatic bone loss. Orthop Rev (Pavia) 2012; 4(1): e14.
[http://dx.doi.org/10.4081/or.2012.e14] [PMID: 22577502]

[23] Childs SG. Stimulators of bone healing. Biologic and biomechanical. Orthop Nurs 2003; 22(6): 421-8.
[http://dx.doi.org/10.1097/00006416-200311000-00010] [PMID: 14705472]

[24] Ghodadra N, Singh K. Recombinant human bone morphogenetic protein-2 in the treatment of bone fractures. Biologics 2008; 2(3): 345-54.
[PMID: 19707367]

[25] Buttaro MA, Costantini J, Comba F, Piccaluga F. The use of femoral struts and impacted cancellous bone allograft in patients with severe femoral bone loss who undergo revision total hip replacement: a three- to nine-year follow-up. J Bone Joint Surg Br 2012; 94(2): 167-72.
[http://dx.doi.org/10.1302/0301-620X.94B2.27296] [PMID: 22323680]

[26] Watson JT, Kuldjanov D. Bone Defects.Limb Lengthening and Reconstruction Surgery. New York: Informa Healthcare 2007; pp. 185-202.

[27] Hernigou P, Poignard A, Beaujean F, Rouard H. Percutaneous autologous bone-marrow grafting for nonunions. Influence of the number and concentration of progenitor cells. J Bone Joint Surg Am 2005; 87(7): 1430-7.
[PMID: 15995108]

[28] Vadalà G, Di Martino A, Tirindelli MC, Denaro L, Denaro V. Use of autologous bone marrow cells concentrate enriched with platelet-rich fibrin on corticocancellous bone allograft for posterolateral multilevel cervical fusion. J Tissue Eng Regen Med 2008; 2(8): 515-20.
[http://dx.doi.org/10.1002/term.121] [PMID: 18972577]

[29] Murawski CD, Kennedy JG. Percutaneous internal fixation of proximal fifth metatarsal jones fractures (Zones II and III) with Charlotte Carolina screw and bone marrow aspirate concentrate: an outcome study in athletes. Am J Sports Med 2011; 39(6): 1295-301.
[http://dx.doi.org/10.1177/0363546510393306] [PMID: 21212308]

[30] Hernigou P, Trousselier M, Roubineau F, *et al.* Local transplantation of bone marrow concentrated granulocytes precursors can cure without antibiotics infected nonunion of polytraumatic patients in absence of bone defect. Int Orthop 2016; 40(11): 2331-8.
[http://dx.doi.org/10.1007/s00264-016-3147-x] [PMID: 26928724]

CHAPTER 6

Management of Osteoarthritis

Mohamed A. Mokhtar[1], Mohamed A. Imam[1,*], Florian Grubhofer[2] and Asser A. Sallam[1]

[1] *Department of Orthopaedics, University of Zurich, Balgrist University Hospital, Switzerland*

[2] *Department of Trauma and Orthopedic Surgery, Suez Canal University Hospitals, Ismailia, Egypt*

Abstract: Mesenchymal stem cells (MSCs) are perceived as an innovative approach to manage osteoarthritis (OA). There are anticipations that MSCs might improve symptoms, function, suppress inflammation and improve cartilage healing. Notwithstanding, the usage of MSCs in the treatment of osteoarthritis needs to be adequately represented, as there are many crucial determinants that should be considered before definitive reliable conclusions concerning the role of MSCs as a treatment option of OA can be drawn.

Keywords: Arthritis, Bone Marrow, Bone Marrow Aspirate Concentrate (BMAC), Osteoarthritis, Stem Cells.

INTRODUCTION

BMAC plays an important role as the main source of growth factors which remain vital in the management of osteoarthritis (OA) because of their anabolic and anti-inflammatory influences. These growth factors, include platelet-derived growth factor (PDGF), transforming growth factor–beta (TGF-β), and bone morphogenetic protein (BMP–2 and BMP-7), which have both anabolic and anti-inflammatory characteristics [1]. Additionally, MSCs have the ability to modulate inflammation, suppress apoptosis, encourage endogenous cell proliferation and repair, and enhance vascularity [2].

* **Corresponding author Mohamed A. Imam:** Department of Trauma and Orthopedic Surgery, Suez Canal University Hospitals, Ismailia, Egypt; The Royal Orthopaedic Hospital, Birmingham, UK; Tel; +44 121 685 4000; Fax: +44 121 685 4100; E-mail: Mohamed.imam@aol.com

CLINICAL IMPLICATIONS OF EXPANDED STEM CELLS IN OSTEOARTHRITIS

A major contention survives about the relative perils of expanded stem cell injections. MSCs that was not cultured in an authorized certified manufacturing practice facility using established culture etiquettes have displayed numerous contingencies including, bacterial contamination, cellular transformation, and/or premature differentiation of cells (Table 1). No recorded side effects connected with MSC transformation, nonetheless, remains a theoretical concern that cells may differentiate or transform into undesired cell types or become oncogenic, especially over the long-term use. To state, there were not any recorded long-term safety predicaments following allogeneic and autologous MSC use. Lately, MSCs were distinguished into multiple subtypes; pro-inflammatory *versus* anti-inflammatory responses based on the activation of toll-like receptors 4 and 3, sequentially, which is expressly applicable for choosing relevant processing manoeuvring targeting the inflammatory diseases [3 - 5]. Detailed analysis of the potential complications is reported in a separate chapter.

Table 1. Sources for mesenchymal stem cells [6].

Tissue type	Advantage	Disadvantage
Bone Marrow	• Good chondrogenic and osteogenic potential • Easy to harvest and exist in large numbers • High proliferative activity	• Risks of harvesting, such as infection and pain
Synovium	• Best chondrogenic potential • High proliferative activity	• Poor osteogenic potential • Only preclinical studies available
Adipose tissue	• Easily harvested • Available in large numbers	• Lower chondrogenic potential, but may be improved through the use of growth factors
Umbilical cord	• No morbidity with collection • Large capacity for *ex vivo* expansion • Full potential to differentiate into chondrogenic, adipogenic, and osteogenic lineages	• Allogenic source • Less well studied

SOME ANIMAL MODELS THAT USE MESENCHYMAL STEM CELLS IN THE MANAGEMENT OF OSTEOARTHRITIS

In one study, collagenase was used to induce OA in the knees of mice; then they were injected with adipose-derived MSCs. These knees showed: decreased thickening of the synovium, decreased osteophytes formation, and reduced articular cartilage damage as compared with the control group [7]. When the knees were injected 14 days after induction of OA, they did not present similar protective capabilities. Therefore, as a conclusion, the early intervention is crucial in modulating OA progression. According to Diekman *et al.* [8] study that used a closed tibial plateau fracture model for inducing posttraumatic arthritis (PTA) in the knees of C57BL/6 mice. Single intra-articular injection of expanded stem cells at the time of fracture is quite enough to guard against post-traumatic arthritis (PTA). On the other hand, Mice in the control group suffered from PTA after 8 weeks from the exposure to the fracture. They observed a rise in the level of cytokines in these MSC-treated mice. These included raised IL-10 level that suggests the presence of an anti-inflammatory effect in the MSC inject. It is worth mentioning that the immune mechanisms differ in murine and human MSCs, consequently, applying this to humans might generate inconsistent outcomes [7, 9].

In a different Model of a rat, 12-weeks old, where partial meniscectomy was done, followed by single intra-articular injection of rat induced rMSCs and human-induced hMSCs. At 2 and 4 weeks mark, there was a nearly comparable incidence of meniscal restoration with both rMSCs and hMSCs, while at 8 weeks mark, the hMSCs showed that it had upper hand in suppressing the progression of OA when compared to the control group.

In a second study, hMSCs were injected in 7 months old guinea pigs with early-onset knee OA around 3 months of age [10]. The study includes 4 groups; a group injected with phosphate buffered saline (PBS), another group with Hyaluronic acid (HA), the third one was injected by PBS and hMSC, and finally, that group injected using hMSCs and HA. Injection of HA+hMSC even if once done, could result in lowering the score of OA and results in partial cartilage repair. These changes were unique enough, so they were absent in the control groups injected with PBS only or HA, rather than those groups injected with PBS and hMSCs.

The effectiveness of MSCs in the treatment of OA was clear evident using the model of induced subchondral defects in the knees of white adult rabbits in New Zealand. It was about the injection of bone marrow or periosteal derived MSCs into the rabbits' knees, the results showed a clear improvement in the macroscopic appearance and histologic scores (Hyaline cartilage) compared with the control group [11]. Having a look at adipose-derived stem cells being injected into the anteromedial compartment of rabbit knees where an anterior cruciate ligament ACL has been transacted. It showed an improved both radiologic and histologic scores when compared to controls.

Also, Goat knees were injected with MSCs at about 6 weeks after total meniscectomy of their medial meniscus and resection of their ACLs. The study displayed an obvious regeneration of the medial meniscus and lesser articular-cartilage damage compared to the control group. On the other hand, sheep knees were also incorporated by injecting MSCs 6 weeks after transection of their ACLs, chondrogenic media induced bone marrow or basal media induced bone marrow MSCs, the chondrogenic induced media showed better results for the cartilage lesions repair, moreover it showed also capabilities to repair some meniscal lesions with meniscus-like tissue. This, it can be concluded that pre-differentiation is a very effective strategy in contrast to the use of undifferentiated MSCs [11, 12].

A trial of intra-articular injection of adipose-derived stromal vascular fraction and bone marrow-derived MSCs 14 days after surgery in knees of horses compared to controls as a guard and treatment of OA. The controls include those injected with a placebo, the results showed that there is no significant effect on pain scores or either radiological or histological examinations. The single beneficial change was the decrease in the levels of prostaglandins E2 in the synovium of the horses 35 days after injection [14].

To sum up, most animal studies were based more on histological evidence rather than functional assessment, making things difficult to translate it clinically on OA patients. No doubt that results will be varied according to the severity of the model, the injury timing and the type of MSCs, also its culture method and for sure its dose [12 - 14].

CLINICAL TRAILS ON HUMAN BEINGS USING EXPANDED MESENCHYMAL STEM CELLS IN THE MANAGEMENT OF OSTEOARTHRITIS

Using autologous MSCs to enhance cartilage regeneration have been used to manage extensive uni-compartmental articular cartilage defects in an arthritic knee; these were done in 12 patients compared with a cell free control group. It was found that both histological findings and arthroscopic examination were all improved, but regarding clinical outcomes, no significant difference. Study was done on 10 patients by injecting expanded stem cells after culturing for 7 days, at 1 year follow up, there were no reported adverse effect either local or systemic. Moreover, patients witnessed statistically significant improvements in pain control using visual analog score (VAS) and Western Ontario and McMaster Universities Arthritis Index (WOMAC) pain scores. In addition to the clear improvements in function capabilities including; increase range of motion, increased walking distance to pain and reduction of patellar crepitus. This was supported also by the MRI findings whereas there were evidence of cartilage repair and extension of this repair to the surrounding tissues, in addition to decreased subchondral bone oedema [15].

In a pilot study includes 4 patients suffering from variable degrees of knee OA ranging from moderate to severe, received bone marrow MSCs intra-articular injection, 6 months follow up results were very satisfactory whereas the walking time before patients suffer pain increased, improvements regarding climbing stairs, knee crepitus and joint swelling. It was worth mentioning that there was no adverse effect reported, also no radiographic changes noted in post-procedure imaging [16].

A study carried by Emadedin *et al.* [17] to evaluate expanded infrapatellar fat pad MSCs injection on 6 female patients with grade IV knee OA according to Kellgren-Lawrence grading system based on radiographs and MRI findings. At one year follow up, nearly all the patients showed improvements in pain control according the VAS and WOMAC pain scores, also they had improved functional capabilities with no reported adverse effects [18, 19].

Twelve patients with knees OA undergone a study where 80-90 ml of bone marrow was aspirated from there iliac bones after applying local anaesthesia and use slight sedation, after 3 weeks as a mean period for cell expansion, the expanded stem cells were collected and then have been injected in the affected knees followed by a period of one-year for follow up. Results were as follows; the procedures themselves (both the marrow collection and the knees injections) were well tolerated by most of the candidates, there were significant improvement in both function and pain control scores measured by VAS and WOMAC scores [20].

Other Sides of the Investigation

Despite current achievements, MSCs being used in the treatment of OA needs to be clearly defined. According to on-going studies listed by Barry and Murphy focusing on use of MSCs in all human body joints affected by OA, like hips, knees and ankles [20]; still present some crucial hurdles that need to be more addressed and detailed prior to a reasoned and reliable conclusion could be drawn regarding the role of MSCs in the treatment of OA.

1. Most of the studies carried focused on the role of expanded stem cells and bone marrow as symptomatic treatments like for improving pain and function scores in knee OA, whilst there is a very little or no evidence that MSCs being intra-articular injected have a role is modifying the course of the disease.
2. It is still unclear which method of administration is the ideal, many studies did not make the comparison between MSCs injections as a scaffold media or

being in suspension [21].

3. Some issues while using MSCs remain controversial as optimal dosage, frequency and number of injections, among most of animal studies and also for the clinical studies on humans, no clear indication of the amount of the initial dose, although it has been suggested by many animal and clinical studies that dose range should be 1 x 106 to 4 x 107 cells per injection [22].

4. The MSCs are being obtained from a various sources (bone marrow, adipose tissue, synovium, and umbilical cord blood or tissues), however, the optimal source is still unclear, most of studies highlighted that they obtain MSCs from marrow or adipose tissues.

5. The studies lack a method to follow the MSCs after injection to know where they end up, for example a clinical imaging study.

6. It is not uncommon for many patients suffering from OA to have either malalignment (varus or valgus knees) or mechanical axis deformities in their affected knees. Therefore, it is crucial to correct such deformities concurrently with the use of MSCs as a treatment for OA. It is also quite important to look for the knee-joint stability as well as the integrity of the menisci, it is certain that surrounding healthy ligaments and musclo-tendinous structures contribute to the proper function of the knee joint [23].

CONSENT FOR PUBLICATION

Not applicable.

CONFLICT OF INTEREST

The authors declare no conflict of interest, financial or otherwise.

ACKNOWLEDGEMENTS

Declared none.

REFERENCES

[1] Carragee EJ, Hurwitz EL, Weiner BK. A critical review of recombinant human bone morphogenetic protein-2 trials in spinal surgery: emerging safety concerns and lessons learned. Spine J 2011; 11(6): 471-91.
[http://dx.doi.org/10.1016/j.spinee.2011.04.023] [PMID: 21729796]

[2] Hall MP, Band PA, Meislin RJ, Jazrawi LM, Cardone DA. Platelet-rich plasma: current concepts and application in sports medicine. J Am Acad Orthop Surg 2009; 17(10): 602-8.
[http://dx.doi.org/10.5435/00124635-200910000-00002] [PMID: 19794217]

[3] Jüni P, Rutjes AW, da Costa BR, Reichenbach S. Viscosupplementation for osteoarthritis of the knee. Ann Intern Med 2013; 158(1): 75.
[http://dx.doi.org/10.7326/0003-4819-158-1-201301010-00020] [PMID: 23277909]

[4] Khoshbin A, Leroux T, Wasserstein D, Marks P, Theodoropoulos J, Ogilvie-Harris D, *et al.* The efficacy of platelet-rich plasma in the treatment of symptomatic knee osteoarthritis: a systematic

review with quantitative synthesis Arthroscopy : the journal of arthroscopic & related surgery : official publication of the Arthroscopy Association of North America and the International Arthroscopy Association 2013;29(12):2037-48
[http://dx.doi.org/10.1016/j.arthro.2013.09.006]

[5]   Mazzocca AD, McCarthy MB, Intravia J, Beitzel K, Apostolakos J, Cote MP, *et al.* An *in vitro* evaluation of the anti-inflammatory effects of platelet-rich plasma, ketorolac, and methylprednisolone. Arthroscopy : the journal of arthroscopic & related surgery : official publication of the Arthroscopy Association of North America and the International Arthroscopy Association 2013;29(4):675-83.

[6]   Hunter DJ. Osteoarthritis. Best Pract Res Clin Rheumatol 2011; 25(6): 801-14.
[http://dx.doi.org/10.1016/j.berh.2011.11.008] [PMID: 22265262]

[7]   Michael JW, Schlüter-Brust KU, Eysel P. The epidemiology, etiology, diagnosis, and treatment of osteoarthritis of the knee. Dtsch Arztebl Int 2010; 107(9): 152-62.
[PMID: 20305774]

[8]   Diekman BO, Wu CL, Louer CR, *et al.* Intra-articular delivery of purified mesenchymal stem cells from C57BL/6 or MRL/MpJ superhealer mice prevents posttraumatic arthritis. Cell Transplant 2013; 22(8): 1395-408.
[http://dx.doi.org/10.3727/096368912X653264] [PMID: 22889498]

[9]   ter Huurne M, Schelbergen R, Blattes R, *et al.* Antiinflammatory and chondroprotective effects of intraarticular injection of adipose-derived stem cells in experimental osteoarthritis. Arthritis Rheum 2012; 64(11): 3604-13.
[http://dx.doi.org/10.1002/art.34626] [PMID: 22961401]

[10]   Sato M, Uchida K, Nakajima H, *et al.* Direct transplantation of mesenchymal stem cells into the knee joints of Hartley strain guinea pigs with spontaneous osteoarthritis. Arthritis Res Ther 2012; 14(1): R31.
[http://dx.doi.org/10.1186/ar3735] [PMID: 22314040]

[11]   Horie M, Choi H, Lee RH, *et al.* Intra-articular injection of human mesenchymal stem cells (MSCs) promote rat meniscal regeneration by being activated to express Indian hedgehog that enhances expression of type II collagen. Osteoarthritis Cartilage 2012; 20(10): 1197-207.
[http://dx.doi.org/10.1016/j.joca.2012.06.002] [PMID: 22750747]

[12]   Toghraie F, Razmkhah M, Gholipour MA, *et al.* Scaffold-free adipose-derived stem cells (ASCs) improve experimentally induced osteoarthritis in rabbits. Arch Iran Med 2012; 15(8): 495-9.
[PMID: 22827787]

[13]   Murphy JM, Fink DJ, Hunziker EB, Barry FP. Stem cell therapy in a caprine model of osteoarthritis. Arthritis Rheum 2003; 48(12): 3464-74.
[http://dx.doi.org/10.1002/art.11365] [PMID: 14673997]

[14]   Frisbie DD, Kisiday JD, Kawcak CE, Werpy NM, McIlwraith CW. Evaluation of adipose-derived stromal vascular fraction or bone marrow-derived mesenchymal stem cells for treatment of osteoarthritis Journal of orthopaedic research : official publication of the Orthopaedic Research Society 2009;27(12):1675-80
[http://dx.doi.org/10.1002/jor.20933]

[15]   Tang QO, Carasco CF, Gamie Z, Korres N, Mantalaris A, Tsiridis E. Preclinical and clinical data for the use of mesenchymal stem cells in articular cartilage tissue engineering. Expert Opin Biol Ther 2012; 12(10): 1361-82.
[http://dx.doi.org/10.1517/14712598.2012.707182] [PMID: 22784026]

[16]   Davatchi F, Abdollahi BS, Mohyeddin M, Shahram F, Nikbin B. Mesenchymal stem cell therapy for knee osteoarthritis. Preliminary report of four patients. Int J Rheum Dis 2011; 14(2): 211-5.
[http://dx.doi.org/10.1111/j.1756-185X.2011.01599.x] [PMID: 21518322]

[17]   Emadedin M, Aghdami N, Taghiyar L, *et al.* Intra-articular injection of autologous mesenchymal stem cells in six patients with knee osteoarthritis. Arch Iran Med 2012; 15(7): 422-8.

[PMID: 22724879]

[18]   Koh YG, Choi YJ. Infrapatellar fat pad-derived mesenchymal stem cell therapy for knee osteoarthritis. Knee 2012; 19(6): 902-7.
[http://dx.doi.org/10.1016/j.knee.2012.04.001] [PMID: 22583627]

[19]   Orozco L, Munar A, Soler R, *et al.* Treatment of knee osteoarthritis with autologous mesenchymal stem cells: a pilot study. Transplantation 2013; 95(12): 1535-41.
[http://dx.doi.org/10.1097/TP.0b013e318291a2da] [PMID: 23680930]

[20]   Barry F, Murphy M. Mesenchymal stem cells in joint disease and repair. Nat Rev Rheumatol 2013; 9(10): 584-94.
[http://dx.doi.org/10.1038/nrrheum.2013.109] [PMID: 23881068]

[21]   Wakitani S, Takaoka K, Hattori T, *et al.* Embryonic stem cells injected into the mouse knee joint form teratomas and subsequently destroy the joint. Rheumatology (Oxford) 2003; 42(1): 162-5.
[http://dx.doi.org/10.1093/rheumatology/keg024] [PMID: 12509630]

[22]   Waterman RS, Tomchuck SL, Henkle SL, Betancourt AM. A new mesenchymal stem cell (MSC) paradigm: polarization into a pro-inflammatory MSC1 or an Immunosuppressive MSC2 phenotype. PLoS One 2010; 5(4): e10088.
[http://dx.doi.org/10.1371/journal.pone.0010088] [PMID: 20436665]

[23]   Zhang W, Nuki G, Moskowitz RW, *et al.* OARSI recommendations for the management of hip and knee osteoarthritis: part III: Changes in evidence following systematic cumulative update of research published through January 2009. Osteoarthritis Cartilage 2010; 18(4): 476-99.
[http://dx.doi.org/10.1016/j.joca.2010.01.013] [PMID: 20170770]

CHAPTER 7

Clinical Applications in Cartilage Pathology

James Holton[1], Mohamed A. Imam[2,3,*], Yasser Elsherbini[4,5] and Martyn Snow[1,2]

[1] *The Royal Orthopaedic Hospital, Birmingham UK*

[2] *University of Birmingham, Birmingham, UK*

[3] *Suez Canal University, Ismailia, Egypt*

[4] *Research and Development, OxCell, OX3 8AT Oxford, UK*

[5] *Institute of Biomedical Engineering, University of Oxford, OX3 7DQ Oxford, UK*

Abstract: Mesenchymal Stem Cells (MSCs) are believed to have multipotent plasticity with the capability to differentiate along multiple cell lineages such as cartilage. This was the foundation on which BMAC has been popularised in the management of cartilage defects. There have been numerous animal models that have shown clear benefit of BMAC to augment healing and improve cartilage repair when compared with traditional cartilage healing techniques; such as micro-fracture. This has been translated into beneficial studies in humans; as diseases of the articular cartilage have such a huge socio-economic burden affecting patient health related quality of life. These pioneering studies have led to a huge increase in the popularity of BMAC as a biological augment. Its key cellular components and growth promoting factors aid tissue regeneration and repair with the potential to produce true hyaline articular. This has clear advantage over the frequently encountered and inferior fibrocartilage from traditional methods of repair, such as microfracture and mosaicoplasty.

Keywords: Bone Marrow, Bone Marrow Aspirate Concentrate (BMAC), Cartilage defects, Osteochondral injuries, Stem Cells.

CARTILAGE AND CARTILAGE DEFECTS

The human articular hyaline cartilage is a specialised connective tissue designed to cope with repetitive loading and provides a low friction surface for ease of motion and reduced wear [1]. The principle cell type is the chondrocyte, arranged within extra-cellular matrix (ECM) [2]. ECM is largely composed of large proteoglycans, proteins and collagens that help retain water, which is the largest component of cartilage [1 - 4]. The collagen component is predominantly of type

---

* **Corresponding author Mohamed A. Imam:** University of Birmingham, Birmingham, UK; Suez Canal University, Ismailia, Egypt; Tel; +44 121 685 4000; Fax: +44 121 685 4100; E-mail: Mohamed.Imam@aol.com

Mohamed A Imam and Martyn Snow (Eds.)

II collagen; yet, there are numerous other subtypes in smaller amounts including I, IV, V, VI, IX and XI [1 - 4]. The articular cartilage is arranged into four distinct zones including superficial, middle, deep and calcified zones [2].

The superficial zone is the interface with the joint and it contains flattened chondrocytes parallel to the joint surface. It has high tensile strength to resist the compressive and sheer forces it is exposed to [1, 3, 4]. The middle zone provides the largest proportion of the cartilage volume collagen content and with its obliquely orientated fibres, provides resistance to compression [4]. However, the deep zone with perpendicularly arranged thick collagen fibres and the largest proteoglycan content provides the greatest resistance to compression [2 - 4]. The calcified zone provides attachment and anchorage to the underlying bone [5].

A unique property of the cartilage is that it does not have a blood supply, lymphatic or nerve supply. It receives its nutrition solely from the synovial fluid of the joint [5]. Its distinct lack of blood supply correlates with its lack of ability to heal as the traditional response to injury is lost [4 - 6]; hence, small defects may propagate enlarging the lesion. Furthermore, lesions that do not cross the calcified zone are limited in healing ability due to the lack of mesenchymal progenitors released from the bone [6]. Nevertheless, if the damage is severe enough to cross the calcified zone and breach the tidemark and cause bleeding, these progenitor cells are released [6, 7]. This allows a healing and regenerative process to begin- although the tissue produced is frequently that of fibrocartilage- which is structurally inferior to the native hyaline articular cartilage [8, 9]. As a result the cartilage is more susceptible to wear and degeneration.

EXPANDED STEM CELLS

The development and clinical application of expanded stem cells has been of huge interest in trauma and orthopaedics as a way to reverse bone and soft tissue injury with the delivery of these multipotent cells [10]. However, one of the main limiting factors to their use is their financial cost associated with harvest and processing. Some sources of stem cells have considerable ethical issues, such as the totipotent embryonic stem cells that require harvest from human embryonic tissue [11, 12]. To overcome the financial and ethical considerations, BMAC has been used as viable source of stem cells. As it is the patients' own cells, it does not elicit an immune response and can be processed at the point of care, at low cost.

Although the bone marrow provides a source of mesenchymal stem cells the true percentage of stem cells is very low at approximately 0.001% of the total volume of bone marrow [14]. This is approximated to 7-30 cells per million nucleated cells [15]. In attempt to increase the concentration the marrow aspirate is concentrated with centrifugation and then it can be used therapeutically [13, 16, 17]. This was discussed in details in a previous chapter.

BMAC USES IN CARTILAGE DEFECTS

In order to avoid the regeneration of fibrocartilage from microfracture and the cost and 2 stage surgery associated with autologous chondrocyte implantation, BMAC has been proposed as a viable alternative to produce hyaline like articular cartilage and ultimately improve outcome. There have been a number of animal studies from rats and rabbits scaling up to larger animals including mini-pig and sheep models [8, 19, 20].

Fortier *et al.* demonstrated that the supplement of BMAC lead to significantly improved cartilage repair when compared with microfracture in an equine model [21]. Large full-thickness cartilage defects were fashioned on the trochlear ridge in 12 horses. The defects were treated with either microfracture alone or combined with BMAC. Second-look was carried out at 12 weeks, and the horses were sacrificed at 8 months. Repair was assessed with use of macroscopic and histological scoring systems as well as with the use quantitative magnetic resonance imaging. The quality of the tissue in the lesions treated with BMAC showed: improved integration into the neighbouring cartilage, greater fill and a superior contoured smoother surface. Despite the clear benefit of using BMAC, the time to develop its therapeutic effect was prolonged. Eight months was the minimum time needed for the maturation of the formed cartilage [21]. This is likely to represent the slow metabolic turnover of chondrocytes and maturation/healing time.

The success of animal studies has allowed translational research into the clinical arena. Gobbi *et al.* reported the outcome of cartilage repair utilizing a single step surgery with BMAC in 15 patients treated for type 4 cartilage defects in the knee at 24 months follow-up [22]. All patients had a mini-arthrotomy and simultaneous implantation with BMAC combined with a collagen matrix. Patients showed significant improvement in Visual analogue scale (VAS), International Knee Documentation Committee score (IKDC) and Knee injury and Osteoarthritis Outcome Score (KOOS) at final follow-up (P < 0.005). Superior outcomes were noticed in patients with solitary cartilage defects and those with small lesions. MRI showed coverage of the lesion with hyaline-like tissue in all patients in accordance with improved clinical results. Hyaline-like histological findings were also reported for all the specimens analysed [22].

To further asses this single step BMAC implantation technique, Gobbi *et al.* conducted a non-randomized prospective comparative trial looking at the outcome of matrix-induced autologous chondrocyte implantation (MACI) *versus* BMAC implantation at a minimum of 3 years post-surgery [23]. They reported no adverse reactions or postoperative surgical complications in either group. Scores were similar for both except for the IKDC score in the BMAC group which was superior (P = 0.015). BMAC showed superior filling of the defects on MRI with 76% in the MACI group compared to 81% the BMAC group [23].

Giannini *et al.* also studied BMAC *versus* open and arthroscopic autologous chondrocyte implantation (ACI) in the talus. They reviewed 81 patients with significant cartilage lesions with an average age of 30 ±8 years [24]. All lesions measured more than 1.5 cm^2 at the time of surgery. For the two arthroscopic repair groups, they utilized a hyaluronic acid membrane to provide support. A second look arthroscopy was undertaken in all patients at 12 months post surgery. For all groups, the average AOFAS score improved from 57.1±17.2 before surgery to 92.6 ±10.5 at an average of 59.5±26.5 months (P<0.0005). There were no significant differences in the change of AOFAS scores between the three groups and histological evaluation emphasized the formation of collagen type II and proteoglycan expression; which is indicative of repair. BMAC provided the advantage of permitting a noticeable decrease in morbidity and costs due to this "one step" BMAC technique.

The use of biomaterials to augment BMAC delivery has also been used in attempt to localize BMAC to the area of concern. A recent study by Enea *et al.*, reported the clinical and histological outcomes of the use of collagen-covered microfracture and BMAC in the management of focal articular cartilage lesions of the knee in nine patients with focal lesions of the femoral condyles. They were managed by arthroscopic microfracture covered with a collagen membrane combined with autologous BMAC. With retrospective assessment, 8/9 (89%) of patients reported significant clinical improvement at an average follow-up of 29 months. 4/9 (44%) patients agreed to undergo a second look arthroscopy and articular biopsy. The macroscopic evaluation of the articular cartilage at one-year follow-up revealed that the repairs appeared almost normal. Histological analysis demonstrated hyaline-like cartilage (1/4), fibrocartilaginous-like cartilage (2/4) and a mixture of both (1/4). The biopsy number is small but shows development of hyaline/hyaline like cartilage regeneration, albeit, in two of the four patients undergoing biopsy. Clearly more significant and long-term analysis is required to assess the histological and functional outcome.

Much of the work looking at cartilage regeneration and repair has focused on focal lesion rather than global areas of degeneration, such as osteoarthritis. Kim *et al.* reviewed 41 patients with diagnosed osteoarthritis and injected them with BMAC [18]. This study found clear beneficial effects, with improved functional quality of life scores and pain scores in patients with osteoarthritis of the knee

[18]. This study highlights the therapeutic potential of BMAC in treating chronic degenerative disease rather than focal sites from damage or injury.

SUMMARY

BMAC has clear potential of being a beneficial and cost effective alternative to autologous chondrocyte implantation and microfracture. Nonetheless, there is a clear need for future research to review the long-term outcomes of BMAC compared to traditional cartilage repair and regenerative techniques.

CONSENT FOR PUBLICATION

Not applicable.

CONFLICT OF INTEREST

The authors declare no conflict of interest, financial or otherwise.

ACKNOWLEDGEMENTS

Declared none.

REFERENCES

[1]   Sophia Fox AJ, Bedi A, Rodeo SA. The basic science of articular cartilage: structure, composition, and function. Sports Health 2009; 1(6): 461-8.
        [http://dx.doi.org/10.1177/1941738109350438] [PMID: 23015907]

[2]   Ramachandran M. Basic Orthopaedic Sciences: The Stanmore Guide (Hodder Arnold Publication). CRC Press; 1 edition (27 Oct. 2006); 304 pages.

[3]   Buckwalter JA, Mankin HJ. Articular cartilage: tissue design and chondrocyte-matrix interactions. Instr Course Lect 1998; 47: 477-86.
        [PMID: 9571449]

[4]   Bhosale AM, Richardson JB. Articular cartilage: structure, injuries and review of management. Br Med Bull 2008; 87: 77-95.
        [http://dx.doi.org/10.1093/bmb/ldn025] [PMID: 18676397]

[5]   Newman AP. Articular cartilage repair. Am J Sports Med 1998; 26(2): 309-24.
        [http://dx.doi.org/10.1177/03635465980260022701] [PMID: 9548130]

[6]   Mankin HJ. The response of articular cartilage to mechanical injury. J Bone Joint Surg Am 1982; 64(3): 460-6.
        [http://dx.doi.org/10.2106/00004623-198264030-00022] [PMID: 6174527]

[7]   Frenkel SR, Di Cesare PE. Degradation and repair of articular cartilage. Front Biosci 1999; 4: D671-85.
        [http://dx.doi.org/10.2741/A464] [PMID: 10525475]

[8]   Im G-I. Endogenous cartilage repair by recruitment of stem cells. Tissue Eng Part B Rev 2015.
        [PMID: 26559963]

[9]   Wang Y, Yuan M, Guo Q-Y, Lu S-B, Peng J. Mesenchymal stem cells for treating articular cartilage defects and osteoarthritis. Cell Transplant 2015; 24(9): 1661-78.

[http://dx.doi.org/10.3727/096368914X683485] [PMID: 25197793]

[10]   Cucchiarini M, Orth P, Rey-Rico A, Venkatesan JK, Madry H. Current perspectives in stem cell research for knee cartilage repair Stem Cells Cloning Adv Appl 2014 Jan;1
[http://dx.doi.org/10.2147/SCCAA.S42880]

[11]   Lee EH, Hui JHP. The potential of stem cells in orthopaedic surgery. J Bone Joint Surg Br 2006; 88(7): 841-51.
[http://dx.doi.org/10.1302/0301-620X.88B7.17305] [PMID: 16798982]

[12]   Dominici M, Le Blanc K, Mueller I, *et al.* Minimal criteria for defining multipotent mesenchymal stromal cells. The International Society for Cellular Therapy position statement. Cytotherapy 2006; 8(4): 315-7.
[http://dx.doi.org/10.1080/14653240600855905] [PMID: 16923606]

[13]   Hyer CF, Berlet GC, Bussewitz BW, Hankins T, Ziegler HL, Philbin TM. Quantitative assessment of the yield of osteoblastic connective tissue progenitors in bone marrow aspirate from the iliac crest, tibia, and calcaneus. J Bone Joint Surg Am 2013; 95(14): 1312-6.
[http://dx.doi.org/10.2106/JBJS.L.01529] [PMID: 23864180]

[14]   Batinić D, Marusić M, Pavletić Z, *et al.* Relationship between differing volumes of bone marrow aspirates and their cellular composition. Bone Marrow Transplant 1990; 6(2): 103-7.
[PMID: 2207448]

[15]   Hernigou P, Mathieu G, Poignard A, Manicom O, Beaujean F, Rouard H. Percutaneous autologous bone-marrow grafting for nonunions. Surgical technique. J Bone Joint Surg Am 2006; 88 (Suppl. 1 Pt 2): 322-7.
[http://dx.doi.org/10.2106/00004623-200609001-00015] [PMID: 16951103]

[16]   Bain BJ. The bone marrow aspirate of healthy subjects. Br J Haematol 1996; 94(1): 206-9.
[http://dx.doi.org/10.1046/j.1365-2141.1996.d01-1786.x] [PMID: 8757536]

[17]   Yamamura R, Yamane T, Hino M, *et al.* Possible automatic cell classification of bone marrow aspirate using the CELL-DYN 4000 automatic blood cell analyzer. J Clin Lab Anal 2002; 16(2): 86-90.
[http://dx.doi.org/10.1002/jcla.10025] [PMID: 11948797]

[18]   Kim J-D, Lee GW, Jung GH, *et al.* Clinical outcome of autologous bone marrow aspirates concentrate (BMAC) injection in degenerative arthritis of the knee. Eur J Orthop Surg Traumatol 2014; 24(8): 1505-11.
[http://dx.doi.org/10.1007/s00590-013-1393-9] [PMID: 24398701]

[19]   Al Faqeh H, Nor Hamdan BMY, Chen HC, Aminuddin BS, Ruszymah BHI. The potential of intra-articular injection of chondrogenic-induced bone marrow stem cells to retard the progression of osteoarthritis in a sheep model. Exp Gerontol 2012; 47(6): 458-64.
[http://dx.doi.org/10.1016/j.exger.2012.03.018] [PMID: 22759409]

[20]   Jung M, Kaszap B, Redöhl A, *et al.* Enhanced early tissue regeneration after matrix-assisted autologous mesenchymal stem cell transplantation in full thickness chondral defects in a minipig model. Cell Transplant 2009; 18(8): 923-32.
[http://dx.doi.org/10.3727/096368909X471297] [PMID: 19523325]

[21]   Fortier LA, Potter HG, Rickey EJ, *et al.* Concentrated bone marrow aspirate improves full-thickness cartilage repair compared with microfracture in the equine model. J Bone Joint Surg Am 2010; 92(10): 1927-37.
[http://dx.doi.org/10.2106/JBJS.I.01284] [PMID: 20720135]

[22]   Gobbi A, Karnatzikos G, Scotti C, Mahajan V, Mazzucco L, Grigolo B. One-step cartilage repair with bone marrow aspirate concentrated cells and collagen matrix in full-thickness knee cartilage lesions: results at 2-year follow-up. Cartilage 2011; 2(3): 286-99.
[http://dx.doi.org/10.1177/1947603510392023] [PMID: 26069587]

[23]   Gobbi A, Chaurasia S, Karnatzikos G, Nakamura N. Matrix-induced autologous chondrocyte

implantation *versus* multipotent stem cells for the treatment of large patellofemoral chondral lesions: a nonrandomized prospective trial. Cartilage 2015; 6(2): 82-97.
[http://dx.doi.org/10.1177/1947603514563597] [PMID: 26069711]

[24]   Giannini S, Buda R, Cavallo M, *et al.* Cartilage repair evolution in post-traumatic osteochondral lesions of the talus: from open field autologous chondrocyte to bone-marrow-derived cells transplantation. Injury 2010; 41(11): 1196-203.
[http://dx.doi.org/10.1016/j.injury.2010.09.028] [PMID: 20934692]

CHAPTER 8

Role of BMAC in Avascular Necrosis

Tomek Kowalski[1], Mohamed A. Imam[1,*], Kuen Chin[2] and Martyn Snow[1]

[1] *The Royal Orthopaedic Hospital, Northfield, Birmingham, UK*

[2] *University Hospitals Birmingham NHS Trust, Birmingham, UK*

Abstract: Avascular necrosis (AVN) is characterized by cell death of trabecular bone leading to bone collapse and subsequent joint destruction. Recently, application of bone marrow derived MSCs has been proposed as adjunctive treatment to core decompression for osteonecrosis of femoral head. There have been several studies, which report that BMAC application results in the improvement of outcomes; nevertheless, it is dependent on the stage of osteonecrosis. Superior outcomes are reported, similar to bone preserving procedures in the pre collapse stages. Additionally, the technique has not been associated with any significant complications. The current results are encouraging, however, more studies are required.

Keywords: Avascular necrosis, Bone Marrow, Bone Marrow Aspirate Concentrate (BMAC), Osteonecrosis, Stem Cells.

INTRODUCTION

Avascular necrosis (AVN) is characterized by cell death of trabecular bone leading to bone collapse. It might be caused by temporary or permanent loss of blood supply to osteocytes with the majority of cases usually preceded by trauma. However, non-traumatic osteonecrosis may be triggered by steroid use, alcohol, sickle cell disease, infection, bone marrow infiltrating diseases, hyperbaric disease and immune factors [1]. AVN most commonly involves the femoral head but also the distal femur, lunate, scaphoid, neck of the talus and proximal humerus [2].

Many methods have been described for the treatment of AVN including non-operative and operative options. Non-operative management includes medications like bisphosphonates, shock wave therapy and electric stimuli. Surgical treatment with *core decompression*, vascularized grafts, osteotomies and joint replacement has been utilised over the years [3].

---

* **Corresponding author Mohamed A. Imam:** The Royal Orthopaedic Hospital, Northfield, Birmingham UK; Tel: +44 121 685 4000; Fax: +44 121 685 4100; E-mail: Mohamed.imam@aol.com

Most recently, there has been a lot of interest in utilizing expanded stem cells (mainly derived from bone marrow) and BMAC in the treatment of AVN.

The proposed effectiveness of adjunctive treatment with these cells may be related to the diminished number of progenitor cells available at the site of osteonecrosis [4] and was first described in the treatment of femoral head necrosis by Hernigou *et al.* [5]. It has been shown that MSCs can provide trophic support to chondrocytes [6, 7] and osteocytes [8, 9] and contribute to tissue regeneration [10].

The outcome of the treatment for AVN is dependent on the stage of osteonecrosis. Several studies demonstrated that the combination of core decompression (CD) with BMAC application might be beneficial in terms of joint preservation in the *pre-collapse stages (I and II)*. Out of the 189 hips, reported by Hernigou and Beaujean [11], treated with CD + BMAC injection in the early stages of AVN-only 9/145 (6.2%) required a total hip replacement at mean of five years compared to 25/44 (56,8%) treated in more advanced stages (after femoral head collapse).

CD and BMAC application in femoral head AVN might be beneficial over CD treatment alone in terms of pain relief. In the study by Gangji *et al.* [12], 18 hips were allocated into two groups, a control of CD *versus* treatment with CD + BMAC; after 24 months, there was a significantly higher reduction in pain in the BMAC group with only one of the hips progressing to stage III in the BMAC group compared with 5 in the control. The same cohort was evaluated in a long-term follow-up at 60 months [13]. Eight of eleven hips treated with CD alone deteriorated and went onto collapse whereas, only 3 out of 13 hips treated with both CD and BMAC progressed to that stage. The authors reported only minor side effects.

Similarly, the clinical outcomes assessed by Harris Hip Score and mean hip survival were superior in a group of 26 hips treated with a combination of CD and BMAC compared with 25 hips treated with CD only in a randomized controlled prospective study by Sen *et al.* [13]. The authors also noted that patients in the group treated with BMAC: had better Harris Hip score, lower oedema, less effusion as well as significantly superior clinical outcome and hip survival.

A novel technique of CD with BMAC and PRP was used to treat early stage femoral head AVN. Martin *et al.* reported this technique [14]; it requires harvesting 2 vials (57 ml each) of bone marrow from the iliac crest, mixing with heparin and centrifuging for 15 min to obtain 2 x 6 ml of BMAC. In addition to that, 120 ml of whole blood is withdrawn and centrifuged to obtain 12 ml of PRP. The combination of BMAC and PRP are applied through a trocar, after core decompression, to the femoral head. Out of the 77 hips treated with this technique, only 16 (21%) deteriorated and required hip replacement. Significant pain relief was reported in 86% of patients; no significant complications were reported.

To address the concern of insufficient number of cells obtained from the iliac crest, Zhao *et al.* [15] proposed autologous implantation of expanded stem cells. These iliac crest bone marrow-derived cultured mononuclear cells, which provided tens of thousands of bone marrow mesenchymal stem cells was used in one hundred recruited patients with early stage AVN. These patients were randomly assigned to a control CD group or a treatment group who were implanted with bone marrow derived expanded stem cells. In the 6-month follow up, only 2 out of 53 patients in the cultured MSC group progressed and required further surgeries compared to 10 out of 44 hips (7 lost in follow up) in the control group who subsequently underwent hip replacement or vascularized bone grafting. The cultured MSC implantation group also had significantly better Harris Hip score; the authors did not report any adverse events in relations to the implantation group.

The safety of BMAC harvesting and its application in AVN cases were investigated in a cohort of 101 patients by Hendrich *et al.* [16]. The study included 37 necrosis of the femoral head, 32 avascular necrosis/bone marrow edema of other joints, 12 non-unions and 20 other defects. Patients were evaluated after a mean of 14 months. Only two patients required further surgeries due to a deterioration of the AVN of the femoral head. However, no further complications were observed: no infections, no excessive new bone formation, no induction of tumor formation and no morbidity due to the bone marrow aspiration from the iliac crest.

SUMMARY

BMAC may be considered a safe adjunctive to surgical treatment in osteonecrosis. There are increasing indications for its use in managing AVN and various orthopaedic procedures [17]. More studies are still required to determine the most effective BMAC preparation and method of application.

CONSENT FOR PUBLICATION

Not applicable.

CONFLICT OF INTEREST

The authors declare no conflict of interest, financial or otherwise.

ACKNOWLEDGEMENTS

Declared none.

REFERENCES

[1]   Assouline-Dayan Y, Chang C, Greenspan A, Shoenfeld Y, Gershwin ME. Pathogenesis and natural history of osteonecrosis. Semin Arthritis Rheum 2002; 32(2): 94-124.
[http://dx.doi.org/10.1053/sarh.2002.33724b] [PMID: 12430099]

[2]   Shah KN, Racine J, Jones LC, Aaron RK. Pathophysiology and risk factors for osteonecrosis. Curr Rev Musculoskelet Med 2015; 8(3): 201-9.
[http://dx.doi.org/10.1007/s12178-015-9277-8] [PMID: 26142896]

[3]   Zalavras CG, Lieberman JR. Osteonecrosis of the femoral head: evaluation and treatment. J Am Acad Orthop Surg 2014; 22(7): 455-64.
[http://dx.doi.org/10.5435/JAAOS-22-07-455] [PMID: 24966252]

[4]   Hernigou P, Beaujean F, Lambotte JC. Decrease in the mesenchymal stem-cell pool in the proximal femur in corticosteroid-induced osteonecrosis. J Bone Joint Surg Br 1999; 81(2): 349-55.
[http://dx.doi.org/10.1302/0301-620X.81B2.8818] [PMID: 10204950]

[5]   Hernigou P. Autologous bone marrow grafting of avascular osteonecrosis before col- lapse. Rev Rhum Engl Ed 1995; 62: 650-1.

[6]   Zuo Q, Cui W, Liu F, Wang Q, Chen Z, Fan W. Co-cultivated mesenchymal stem cells support chondrocytic differentiation of articular chondrocytes. Int Orthop 2013; 37(4): 747-52.
[http://dx.doi.org/10.1007/s00264-013-1782-z] [PMID: 23354690]

[7]   Halvorsen YD, Franklin D, Bond AL, *et al.* Extracellular matrix mineralization and osteoblast gene expression by human adipose tissue-derived stromal cells. Tissue Eng 2001; 7(6): 729-41.
[http://dx.doi.org/10.1089/107632701753337681] [PMID: 11749730]

[8]   Kim BS, Kim JS, Chung YS, *et al.* Growth and osteogenic differentiation of alveolar human bone marrow-derived mesenchymal stem cells on chitosan/hydroxyapatite composite fabric. J Biomed Mater Res A 2013; 101(6): 1550-8.
[http://dx.doi.org/10.1002/jbm.a.34456] [PMID: 23135904]

[9]   Crisan M, Corselli M, Chen WC, Péault B. Perivascular cells for regenerative medicine. J Cell Mol Med 2012; 16(12): 2851-60.
[http://dx.doi.org/10.1111/j.1582-4934.2012.01617.x] [PMID: 22882758]

[10] Hernigou P, Beaujean F. Treatment of osteonecrosis with autologous bone marrow grafting. Clin Orthop Relat Res 2002; (405): 14-23.
[http://dx.doi.org/10.1097/00003086-200212000-00003] [PMID: 12461352]

[11] Gangji V, Hauzeur JP, Matos C, De Maertelaer V, Toungouz M, Lambermont M. Treatment of osteonecrosis of the femoral head with implantation of autologous bone-marrow cells. A pilot study. J Bone Joint Surg Am 2004; 86-A(6): 1153-60.
[http://dx.doi.org/10.2106/00004623-200406000-00006] [PMID: 15173287]

[12] Gangji V, De Maertelaer V, Hauzeur JP. Autologous bone marrow cell implantation in the treatment of non-traumatic osteonecrosis of the femoral head: Five year follow-up of a prospective controlled study. Bone 2011; 49(5): 1005-9.
[http://dx.doi.org/10.1016/j.bone.2011.07.032] [PMID: 21821156]

[13] Sen RK, Tripathy SK, Aggarwal S, Marwaha N, Sharma RR, Khandelwal N. Early results of core decompression and autologous bone marrow mononuclear cells instillation in femoral head osteonecrosis: a randomized control study. J Arthroplasty 2012; 27(5): 679-86.
[http://dx.doi.org/10.1016/j.arth.2011.08.008] [PMID: 22000577]

[14]   Martin JR, Houdek MT, Sierra RJ. Use of concentrated bone marrow aspirate and platelet rich plasma during minimally invasive decompression of the femoral head in the treatment of osteonecrosis. Croat Med J 2013; 54(3): 219-24.
[http://dx.doi.org/10.3325/cmj.2013.54.219] [PMID: 23771751]

[15]   Zhao D, Cui D, Wang B, *et al.* Treatment of early stage osteonecrosis of the femoral head with autologous implantation of bone marrow-derived and cultured mesenchymal stem cells. Bone 2012; 50(1): 325-30.
[http://dx.doi.org/10.1016/j.bone.2011.11.002] [PMID: 22094904]

[16]   Hendrich C, Franz E, Waertel G, Krebs R, Jäger M. Safety of autologous bone marrow aspiration concentrate transplantation: initial experiences in 101 patients. Orthop Rev (Pavia) 2009; 1(2): e32.
[http://dx.doi.org/10.4081/or.2009.e32] [PMID: 21808691]

[17]   Imam MA, Mahmoud SSS, Holton J, Abouelmaati D, Elsherbini Y, Snow M. A systematic review of the concept and clinical applications of Bone Marrow Aspirate Concentrate in Orthopaedics 2017; SICOT J, 3, 17
[http://dx.doi.org/10.1051/sicotj/2017007]

CHAPTER 9

Bone Marrow Aspirate Concentrate in Nerve and Spinal Cord Injury

Asser A. Sallam[1,*], Mohamed A. Imam[2] and Ali Narvani[3]

[1] *Department of Trauma and Orthopedic Surgery, Suez Canal University Hospitals, Ismailia, Egypt*

[2] *The Royal Orthopaedic Hospital, Birmingham, B31 2AP, UK; Suez Canal University Hospitals, Ismailia, 41111, Egypt*

[3] *Ashford and St Peter's NHS Trust, Chertsey, Surrey, UK*

Abstract: Nerve injuries either peripheral or central are extremely frequent in clinical practice. The impairment of sensory and motor functions may have distressing effects on the social and professional activities of these patients, most of whom are young and may acquire life-long disabilities. The extent of disability and patient suffering after Spinal Cord Injuries (SCI), as well as the high cost of care, continues to motivate research into effective interventions. Nerve surgery is aimed at motor and sensory reinnervation, but often a deficit in the functionality remains. As cell therapy and tissue engineering have been receiving a great deal of attention in recent decades, and are widely used in different areas, Therefore, the utilization of bone marrow aspirate concentrate in peripheral nerve repair techniques as well as after spinal cord injury is tried in order to optimize the regeneration process. In this chapter, we will discuss the evidence in the literature regarding the clinical and experimental application of bone marrow aspirate concentrate as a major source of mesenchymal stem cells in treatment of peripheral nerve and spinal cord injuries.

Keywords: Bone Marrow Aspirate Concentrate (BMAC), Expanded stem cells, Mesenchymal Stem Cells (MSCs), Nerve Injury, Spinal cord injury, Spinal cord transection.

1.1. PERIPHERAL NERVE INJURY

Injuries of peripheral nerves affect about 2.8% of trauma patients [1]. Even a digital nerve injury resulting from a minor finger trauma may induce hand dysfunction. The injury negatively influences the patient's professional life and leisure activities as a result of functional impairment. Furthermore, the principal part of the total cost of nerve injuries is due to productivity loss in the form of sick

---

* **Corresponding author Asser A. Sallam:** Department of Trauma and Orthopedic Surgery, Suez Canal University Hospitals, Ismailia, Egypt; Tel: +20 109 52772120; E-mail: assersallam@hotmail.com

Mohamed A Imam and Martyn Snow (Eds.)

leave. This reflects the demographics of the injury, with the majority of patients being young and of working age. An effective and accurately timed management of peripheral nerve injuries is essential to accomplish the best clinical and functional outcomes [2].

Being delicate structures, peripheral nerve trunks consist of the nerve cell, body, axons and other cellular components as well as intraneural blood vessels that might be disturbed by trauma [3].

Despite the capability of peripheral nerves to regenerate and re-innervate distal targets, frustrating functional outcomes persist. The level and mechanism of the injury, the type and degree of the injury, the timing of the repair, and patient factors all contribute to the outcome after nerve injury [4, 5]. Moreover, the hand skill and policies applied by the peripheral nerve surgeons can have a spectacular effect. Microsurgical nerve repair possesses significant advantages and have led to better outcomes after peripheral nerve reconstructive surgeries [5].

In more severe injuries, large gap or lengthy scar within the nerve precludes axonal regeneration [6]. In these situations when direct end-to-end neurorrhaphy is impossible, autologous nerve grafting is considered to be the gold standard of repair. However, recovery is restricted by inadequate and non-specific regeneration with variable functional and clinical outcomes [6, 7]. Scarring, poor blood supply and the necessity of two procedures at different sites are the main limiting factors of peripheral nerve regeneration. Additionally, patients are concerned about the consequent donor site morbidity [8, 9].

Entubulation is an available and widely used repair technique. The divided nerve stumps are introduced and secured inside a biologic or synthetic nerve conduit, aiming to provide a favorable environment for regeneration [8], protect the nerve from the possible surrounding scaring and avoid formation of painful neuroma [10]. Entubulation can be adjusted by the adding neurotrophic factors [11, 12]. The concentration of these factors is critical to advance axonal regeneration, and if the conduit size increases, regeneration is inhibited. Moore *et al.* suggested that the nerve conduits should be utilized only for gaps shorter than 3 cm and to repair noncritical small sensory nerves like digital nerves [13].

Tissue engineering and cell therapy recently offer a therapeutic option to enhance regeneration of peripheral nerve [14]. Cell transplantation is an example of these strategies. It aimed at formation of a suitable microenvironment to enhance tissue regeneration.

Stem cells are considered as undifferentiated precursor cells that have the ability to differentiate into multiple lineages [15]. Expanded stem cells obtained from adult cerebral tissue as well as embryonic stem cells are able to undergo neuronal differentiation not only *in vitro*, but also *in vivo*. However, the unavailability of these cells limits their use in clinical practice [16, 17].

Bone marrow offers a rich source of mesenchymal stem cells [18 - 21]. Adult bone marrow-derived cells are multipotent, possessing the capability of differentiation into mesodermal cell lineages [22]. Several studies have revealed that these cells also have the potential for *in vitro* neuronal differentiation. Therefore, they can be utilized in repair of peripheral nerves [23 - 27].

Experimental studies in rodents [28 - 30], rabbits [31] and primates [32] have proven the competence of these cells in improving functional outcomes after peripheral nerve repair. The use of bone marrow mesenchymal cells in combination with bio-absorbable tubes increases axonal regeneration and functional recovery of sciatic nerve in mice [33]. Bone marrow mesenchymal cells can enhance the peripheral nerve regeneration through the direct release of neurotrophic factors, as well as the indirect stimulation of Schwann cells [34].

There is clinical evidence confirming the use of bone marrow mesenchymal cells as an efficient adjuvant therapy in peripheral nerve repair. Comparing the entubulation technique with and without adding bone marrow mononuclear cells in 44 patients suffering median or ulnar nerve injuries, it was reported that lesions managed by these cells presented better results in the regeneration process than conventional entubulation [11]. Nevertheless, bone marrow mesenchymal cells have some limitations. The harvesting technique is painful as these cells are obtained through the application of epidural or general anesthesia. Also, the acquired cells frequently fail to reach the needed number [57].

Additionally, Hogendoorn *et al.* assessed the safety and regenerative potential of autologous Bone Marrow Mesenchymal Stem Cells (BMSCs) injection in partially denervated biceps in patients with traumatic brachial plexus injuries. They reported no donor or recipient sites morbidity. Following injection, there was a 52% diminution in muscle fibrosis, an 80% increase in myofibre diameter, a 50% increase in satellite cells and an 83% increase in capillary-to-myofibre ratio. Similarly, CT analysis verified a 48% reduction in mean density of the muscle. Analysis of motor unit presented a mean increase of amplitude, duration and number of phases. These results imply the importance of BMSCs injection in partially denervated muscle in patients suffering brachial plexus palsy as it is safe and enhances muscle regeneration and reinnervation.

A recent review [35] comparing the results of using either concentrated and culture-expanded BMSCs *versus* native whole bone marrow aspirate, revealed that currently applied concentration methods do not attain sufficient concentration or number of mesenchymal stem cells from bone marrow aspirate. In addition, it was revealed that the cells show a more rapid proliferation rate at lower seeding numbers. Therefore, a rapid expansion to attain enough cells can be achieved by using smaller cell numbers. There is still a scarcity of data in the literature as regard to the concentration of mesenchymal stem cells at sites of nerve injury.

Spinal Cord Injury

Adult bone marrow delivers plenty of progenitor cells derived from hematopoietic as well as nonhematopoietic stem cells (*e.g.* bone, cartilage, muscle, glia, neurons). They possess the ability to secrete interleukins and other trophic factors [36 - 38], and to replace damaged cells; thus enabling neural regeneration, and consequently functional recovery following spinal cord injury (SCI). Acutely isolated bone marrow cells can be transplanted into patients immediately after harvesting and without expansion in cell culture leading to extensive remyelination [39 - 41].

Chopp *et al*. [42] tested the hypothesis that expanded stem cells transplantation into the contused spinal cord encourages functional outcome in rats. Expanded stem cells were injected into the spinal cord one week following injury and functional outcomes were followed-up on a weekly basis for five weeks. The findings indicate significant improvement in motor power in animals treated with expanded stem cells transplantation compared to control animals. Scattered cells derived from expanded stem cells expressed neural protein markers.

Another study described the effects of expanded stem cells utilization in rats with a balloon-induced spinal cord compression lesion [43] and found that animals with SCI treated by expanded stem cells regained better sensory recovery of hind limb than controls injected with saline. An increase in the spared white matter was observed. Five weeks after SCI, MR images of the spinal cords revealed dark hypointense areas indicating the lesions populated by grafted expanded stem cells. Histological analysis confirmed many iron-containing and PKH 26-positive cells in the lesion site.

Other experimental studies have emphasized that expanded stem cells transplantation in treating spinal cord injury has shown some therapeutic effects. Chen *et al*. [28] investigated the effects of bone marrow mesenchymal stem-cell transplantation (BMSCs) in repairing acute spinal cord damage in rats and reported that motor functions of animals with spinal cord injury significantly improved two weeks following BMSCs transplantation. Histological analysis showed that edema was reduced at the seventh day, inflammatory cell infiltration decreased, vacuolar degeneration improved, the morphology of nerve cells appeared normal, and intracellular structures were evenly arranged. The recovery of nerve cells and structural arrangement was observed by 15 days as compared to tissues examined 7 days post transplantation, indicating that BMSCs transplantation into the area of spinal cord injury can encourage regeneration of the injured spinal cord. This experiment also demonstrated that BMSCs can enter the blood-spinal cord barrier and migrate to the injured spinal cord. The migratory BMSCs reached their target area by day 15 post transplantation; furthermore, surviving cells were expressing the neuronal marker, neuron-specific protein, indicating that BMSCs can migrate to the injured area of the spinal cord utilizing cell-cell contact mechanisms, and promote repair by transforming into neurons.

In clinical practice, the utilization of BMSCs in both incomplete and complete SCI in human has been described [44]. Despite the variability of time to intervention in published research, the majority of the literature recommends early BMSCs intervention in order to encourage better neurologic improvement [45 - 47]. Bhanot [48] explained that the chemokine signals in chronic SCI are too weak to direct stem cells toward the site of injury.

Most available studies also describe the mechanism of spinal injury as blunt trauma, penetrating trauma, or ischemic or iatrogenic SCI. The majority of published studies classify patients according to the American Spinal Injury Association (ASIA) impairment scale [49]. Studies in patients with incomplete injuries demonstrate greater variation in the degree of recovery and greater probability of a positive clinical outcome [44], in contrast to patients with complete injuries [50, 51]. Because of the possibility of spontaneous recovery, injuries graded B and C on the ASIA scale are not typically reported in high-quality articles [49]. Chernykh *et al.* [52] demonstrated that greater motor and sensory recovery is associated with injury to the cervical compared with injury to the thoracic spinal cord. Other studies have reported that injuries to the thoracic spinal cord display better response to bone marrow therapy than injuries to the cervical spinal cord [45].

A recent clinical study was carried out by Dai *et al.* [53] who investigated the treatment of complete and chronic cervical SCI by autologous BMSCs. Forty patients were randomized to either BMSCs transplantation or control. Significant improvements in motor function, light touch, pin-prick sensation, and residual urine volume were observed in 10 of the patients who received BMSCs therapy. Furthermore, 9 patients had changes in their functional scores. The control group did not show any functional improvement.

Similarly, Jiang *et al.* [54] treated 20 patients with SCI with autologous bone BMSCs. Improvement was noted 30 days postintervention in 15 patients in sensory, motor, and autonomic nerve function as evaluated by ASIA scale.

Karamouzian *et al.* [55] investigated the possible side effects or risks associated with BMSCs therapy in subacute thoracic SCI. The BMSCs were introduced into the site of injury through a lumbar puncture, and patients were followed up for about 1-2 years. Although a non-significant functional recovery was observed, no complications were reported in either the experimental or the control group.

Park *et al.* [56] assessed the long-term outcome of BMSCs therapy in patients who received 3 injections every 4-week. Improvement of motor power of upper extremities was achieved in 6/10 patients; of these, 3 improved in activities of daily living. MRI illustrated a reduction in cavity size and fiber-like low-signal intensity streaks.

As stated previously, BMSCs control inflammatory and immune responses and encourage the motor recovery following SCI. Yet, the influence of BMSCs therapy on central neuropathic pain remain unclear. Watanabe *et al.* [57] studied the results of BMSCs transplantation on pain hypersensitivity in mice underwent a spinal cord contusion. BMSCs transplantation on the third day postinjury achieved significant improvement of motor power and relieved hypersensitivities, induced by SCI, to mechanical and thermal stimuli. These findings support the utilization of BMSCs in SCI management. Moreover, they propose that BMSCs relieve the neuropathic pain by several mechanisms that include neuronal sparing and rebuilding of the disturbed blood spinal cord barrier, mediated through modulation of the of microglia and macrophages activity.

CONSENT FOR PUBLICATION

Not applicable.

CONFLICT OF INTEREST

The authors declare no conflict of interest, financial or otherwise.

ACKNOWLEDGEMENTS

Declared none.

REFERENCES

[1]   Noble J, Munro CA, Prasad VS, Midha R. Analysis of upper and lower extremity peripheral nerve injuries in a population of patients with multiple injuries. J Trauma 1998; 45(1): 116-22.
[http://dx.doi.org/10.1097/00005373-199807000-00025] [PMID: 9680023]

[2]   Rosberg HE, Carlsson KS, Hojgard S, *et al.* Injury to the human median and ulnar nerves in the forearm--analysis of costs for treatment and rehabilitation of 69 patients in southern Sweden. J Hand Surg Am 2005; 30(1): 35-9.
[http://dx.doi.org/10.1016/J.JHSB.2004.09.003] [PMID: 15680553]

[3] Dahlin LB. Techniques of peripheral nerve repair Scandinavian journal of surgery: SJS: official organ for the Finnish Surgical Society and the Scandinavian Surgical Society; 2008; 97(4):310-316
[http://dx.doi.org/10.1177/145749690809700407]

[4] Mackinnon SE, Roque B, Tung TH. Median to radial nerve transfer for treatment of radial nerve palsy. Case report. J Neurosurg 2007; 107(3): 666-71.
[http://dx.doi.org/10.3171/JNS-07/09/0666] [PMID: 17886570]

[5] Dvali L, Mackinnon S. The role of microsurgery in nerve repair and nerve grafting. Hand Clin 2007; 23(1): 73-81.
[http://dx.doi.org/10.1016/j.hcl.2007.02.003] [PMID: 17478254]

[6] Kline DG, Kim D, Midha R, Harsh C, Tiel R. Management and results of sciatic nerve injuries: a 24-year experience. J Neurosurg 1998; 89(1): 13-23.
[http://dx.doi.org/10.3171/jns.1998.89.1.0013] [PMID: 9647167]

[7] Midha R. Nerve transfers for severe brachial plexus injuries: a review. Neurosurg Focus 2004; 16(5): E5.
[http://dx.doi.org/10.3171/foc.2004.16.5.6] [PMID: 15174825]

[8] de Olivera A, Pierucci A, de Brito P. Peripheral nerve regeneration through the nerve tubulization technique. Braz J Morphol Sci 2004; 21(4): 225-31.

[9] Ichihara S, Inada Y, Nakamura T. Artificial nerve tubes and their application for repair of peripheral nerve injury: an update of current concepts. Injury 2008; 39 (Suppl. 4): 29-39.
[http://dx.doi.org/10.1016/j.injury.2008.08.029] [PMID: 18804584]

[10] Pierucci A, Faria AM, Pimentel ER, et al. Effects of aggrecan on schwann cell migration in vitro and nerve regeneration in vivo. Braz J Morphol Sci 2004; 21(3): 125-30.

[11] Braga-Silva J, Gehlen D, Padoin AV, Machado DC, Garicochea B, Costa da Costa J. Can local supply of bone marrow mononuclear cells improve the outcome from late tubular repair of human median and ulnar nerves? J Hand Surg Eur Vol 2008; 33(4): 488-93.
[http://dx.doi.org/10.1177/1753193408090401] [PMID: 18687837]

[12] Sariguney Y, Yavuzer R, Elmas C, Yenicesu I, Bolay H, Atabay K. Effect of platelet-rich plasma on peripheral nerve regeneration. J Reconstr Microsurg 2008; 24(3): 159-67.
[http://dx.doi.org/10.1055/s-2008-1076752] [PMID: 18452111]

[13] Moore AM, Kasukurthi R, Magill CK, Farhadi HF, Borschel GH, Mackinnon SE. Limitations of conduits in peripheral nerve repairs. Hand (N Y) 2009; 4(2): 180-6.
[http://dx.doi.org/10.1007/s11552-008-9158-3] [PMID: 19137378]

[14] Sebben AD, Lichtenfels M, da Silva JL. Silva JLBd. Peripheral nerve regeneration: cell therapy and neurotrophic factors. Rev Bras Ortop 2015; 46(6): 643-9.
[PMID: 27027067]

[15] Lemischka IR. Stem cell biology: a view toward the future. Ann N Y Acad Sci 2005; 1044: 132-8.
[http://dx.doi.org/10.1196/annals.1349.017] [PMID: 15958706]

[16] Safford KM, Hicok KC, Safford SD, et al. Neurogenic differentiation of murine and human adipose-derived stromal cells. Biochem Biophys Res Commun 2002; 294(2): 371-9.
[http://dx.doi.org/10.1016/S0006-291X(02)00469-2] [PMID: 12051722]

[17] Zhang F, Blain B, Beck J, et al. Autogenous venous graft with one-stage prepared Schwann cells as a conduit for repair of long segmental nerve defects. J Reconstr Microsurg 2002; 18(4): 295-300.
[http://dx.doi.org/10.1055/s-2002-30186] [PMID: 12022035]

[18] Evans GR, Brandt K, Katz S, et al. Bioactive poly(L-lactic acid) conduits seeded with Schwann cells for peripheral nerve regeneration. Biomaterials 2002; 23(3): 841-8.
[http://dx.doi.org/10.1016/S0142-9612(01)00190-9] [PMID: 11774850]

[19] Galla TJ, Vedecnik SV, Halbgewachs J, Steinmann S, Friedrich C, Stark GB. Fibrin/Schwann cell

matrix in poly-epsilon-caprolactone conduits enhances guided nerve regeneration. Int J Artif Organs 2004; 27(2): 127-36.
[http://dx.doi.org/10.1177/039139880402700208] [PMID: 15068007]

[20]   Diniz D, Avelino D. International perspective on embryonic stem cell research. Rev Saude Publica 2009; 43(3): 541-7.
[http://dx.doi.org/10.1590/S0034-89102009000300019] [PMID: 19377751]

[21]   Lo B, Parham L. Ethical issues in stem cell research. Endocr Rev 2009; 30(3): 204-13.
[http://dx.doi.org/10.1210/er.2008-0031] [PMID: 19366754]

[22]   Abdallah BM, Kassem M. Human mesenchymal stem cells: from basic biology to clinical applications. Gene Ther 2008; 15(2): 109-16.
[http://dx.doi.org/10.1038/sj.gt.3303067] [PMID: 17989700]

[23]   Ohta M, Suzuki Y, Noda T, *et al.* Implantation of neural stem cells *via* cerebrospinal fluid into the injured root. Neuroreport 2004; 15(8): 1249-53.
[http://dx.doi.org/10.1097/01.wnr.0000129998.72184.e1] [PMID: 15167543]

[24]   Tohill M, Mantovani C, Wiberg M, Terenghi G. Rat bone marrow mesenchymal stem cells express glial markers and stimulate nerve regeneration. Neurosci Lett 2004; 362(3): 200-3.
[http://dx.doi.org/10.1016/j.neulet.2004.03.077] [PMID: 15158014]

[25]   Dezawa M, Hoshino M, Nabeshima Y, Ide C. Marrow stromal cells: implications in health and disease in the nervous system. Curr Mol Med 2005; 5(7): 723-32.
[http://dx.doi.org/10.2174/156652405774641070] [PMID: 16305495]

[26]   Keilhoff G, Goihl A, Stang F, Wolf G, Fansa H. Peripheral nerve tissue engineering: autologous Schwann cells *vs.* transdifferentiated mesenchymal stem cells. Tissue Eng 2006; 12(6): 1451-65.
[http://dx.doi.org/10.1089/ten.2006.12.1451] [PMID: 16846343]

[27]   Montzka K, Lassonczyk N, Tschöke B, *et al.* Neural differentiation potential of human bone marrow-derived mesenchymal stromal cells: misleading marker gene expression. BMC Neurosci 2009; 10: 16.
[http://dx.doi.org/10.1186/1471-2202-10-16] [PMID: 19257891]

[28]   Chen X, Wang XD, Chen G, Lin WW, Yao J, Gu XS. Study of *in vivo* differentiation of rat bone marrow stromal cells into schwann cell-like cells. Microsurgery 2006; 26(2): 111-5.
[http://dx.doi.org/10.1002/micr.20184] [PMID: 16453290]

[29]   Yang Y, Yuan X, Ding F, *et al.* Repair of rat sciatic nerve gap by a silk fibroin-based scaffold added with bone marrow mesenchymal stem cells. Tissue Eng Part A 2011; 17(17-18): 2231-44.
[http://dx.doi.org/10.1089/ten.tea.2010.0633] [PMID: 21542668]

[30]   Goel RK, Suri V, Suri A, *et al.* Effect of bone marrow-derived mononuclear cells on nerve regeneration in the transection model of the rat sciatic nerve Journal of clinical neuroscience : official journal of the Neurosurgical Society of Australasia 2009; 16(9):1211-1217
[http://dx.doi.org/10.1016/j.jocn.2009.01.031]

[31]   Choi BH, Zhu SJ, Kim BY, Huh JY, Lee SH, Jung JH. Transplantation of cultured bone marrow stromal cells to improve peripheral nerve regeneration. Int J Oral Maxillofac Surg 2005; 34(5): 537-42.
[http://dx.doi.org/10.1016/j.ijom.2004.10.017] [PMID: 16053875]

[32]   Wang D, Liu XL, Zhu JK, *et al.* Bridging small-gap peripheral nerve defects using acellular nerve allograft implanted with autologous bone marrow stromal cells in primates. Brain Res 2008; 1188: 44-53.
[http://dx.doi.org/10.1016/j.brainres.2007.09.098] [PMID: 18061586]

[33]   Oliveira JT, Almeida FM, Biancalana A, *et al.* Mesenchymal stem cells in a polycaprolactone conduit enhance median-nerve regeneration, prevent decrease of creatine phosphokinase levels in muscle, and improve functional recovery in mice. Neuroscience 2010; 170(4): 1295-303.
[http://dx.doi.org/10.1016/j.neuroscience.2010.08.042] [PMID: 20800664]

[34] Wang J, Ding F, Gu Y, Liu J, Gu X. Bone marrow mesenchymal stem cells promote cell proliferation and neurotrophic function of Schwann cells *in vitro* and *in vivo*. Brain Res 2009; 1262: 7-15.
[http://dx.doi.org/10.1016/j.brainres.2009.01.056] [PMID: 19368814]

[35] Hauser R, Eteshola E. Rationale for using direct bone marrow aspirate as a proliferant for regenerative injection therapy (prolotherapy). Open Stem Cell J 2013; 4: 7-14.
[http://dx.doi.org/10.2174/1876893801304010007]

[36] Eaves CJ, Cashman JD, Kay RJ, *et al.* Mechanisms that regulate the cell cycle status of very primitive hematopoietic cells in long-term human marrow cultures. II. Analysis of positive and negative regulators produced by stromal cells within the adherent layer. Blood 1991; 78(1): 110-7.
[PMID: 1712638]

[37] Majumdar MK, Thiede MA, Mosca JD, Moorman M, Gerson SL. Phenotypic and functional comparison of cultures of marrow-derived mesenchymal stem cells (MSCs) and stromal cells. J Cell Physiol 1998; 176(1): 57-66.
[http://dx.doi.org/10.1002/(SICI)1097-4652(199807)176:1<57::AID-JCP7>3.0.CO;2-7] [PMID: 9618145]

[38] Bjorklund LM, Sánchez-Pernaute R, Chung S, *et al.* Embryonic stem cells develop into functional dopaminergic neurons after transplantation in a Parkinson rat model. Proc Natl Acad Sci USA 2002; 99(4): 2344-9.
[http://dx.doi.org/10.1073/pnas.022438099] [PMID: 11782534]

[39] Sasaki M, Honmou O, Akiyama Y, Uede T, Hashi K, Kocsis JD. Transplantation of an acutely isolated bone marrow fraction repairs demyelinated adult rat spinal cord axons. Glia 2001; 35(1): 26-34.
[http://dx.doi.org/10.1002/glia.1067] [PMID: 11424189]

[40] Akiyama Y, Radtke C, Kocsis JD. Remyelination of the rat spinal cord by transplantation of identified bone marrow stromal cells. J Neurosci : the official journal of the Society for Neuroscience 2002; 22(15):6623-6630.

[41] Inoue M, Honmou O, Oka S, Houkin K, Hashi K, Kocsis JD. Comparative analysis of remyelinating potential of focal and intravenous administration of autologous bone marrow cells into the rat demyelinated spinal cord. Glia 2003; 44(2): 111-8.
[http://dx.doi.org/10.1002/glia.10285] [PMID: 14515327]

[42] Chopp M, Zhang XH, Li Y, *et al.* Spinal cord injury in rat: treatment with bone marrow stromal cell transplantation. Neuroreport 2000; 11(13): 3001-5.
[http://dx.doi.org/10.1097/00001756-200009110-00035] [PMID: 11006983]

[43] Urdzíková L, Jendelová P, Glogarová K, Burian M, Hájek M, Syková E. Transplantation of bone marrow stem cells as well as mobilization by granulocyte-colony stimulating factor promotes recovery after spinal cord injury in rats. J Neurotrauma 2006; 23(9): 1379-91.
[http://dx.doi.org/10.1089/neu.2006.23.1379] [PMID: 16958589]

[44] Kishk NA, Gabr H, Hamdy S, *et al.* Case control series of intrathecal autologous bone marrow mesenchymal stem cell therapy for chronic spinal cord injury. Neurorehabil Neural Repair 2010; 24(8): 702-8.
[http://dx.doi.org/10.1177/1545968310369801] [PMID: 20660620]

[45] Kumar AA, Kumar SR, Narayanan R, *et al.* Autologous bone marrow derived mononuclear cell therapy for spinal cord injury: A phase I/II clinical safety and primary efficacy data. Experimental and clinical transplantation : official journal of the Middle East Society for Organ Transplantation 2009; 7(4):241-248.

[46] Fehlings MG, Vaccaro A, Wilson JR, *et al.* Early *versus* delayed decompression for traumatic cervical spinal cord injury: results of the Surgical Timing in Acute Spinal Cord Injury Study (STASCIS). PLoS One 2012; 7(2): e32037.
[http://dx.doi.org/10.1371/journal.pone.0032037] [PMID: 22384132]

[47]   Chikuda H, Ohtsu H, Ogata T, *et al.* Optimal treatment for spinal cord injury associated with cervical canal stenosis (OSCIS): a study protocol for a randomized controlled trial comparing early *versus* delayed surgery. Trials 2013; 14: 245.
[http://dx.doi.org/10.1186/1745-6215-14-245] [PMID: 23924165]

[48]   Bhanot Y, Rao S, Ghosh D, Balaraju S, Radhika CR, Satish Kumar KV. Autologous mesenchymal stem cells in chronic spinal cord injury. Br J Neurosurg 2011; 25(4): 516-22.
[http://dx.doi.org/10.3109/02688697.2010.550658] [PMID: 21749185]

[49]   Harrop JS, Hashimoto R, Norvell D, *et al.* Evaluation of clinical experience using cell-based therapies in patients with spinal cord injury: a systematic review. J Neurosurg Spine 2012; 17(1) (Suppl.): 230-46.
[http://dx.doi.org/10.3171/2012.5.AOSPINE12115] [PMID: 22985383]

[50]   Burns AS, Lee BS, Ditunno JF Jr, Tessler A. Patient selection for clinical trials: the reliability of the early spinal cord injury examination. J Neurotrauma 2003; 20(5): 477-82.
[http://dx.doi.org/10.1089/089771503765355540] [PMID: 12803979]

[51]   Kirshblum S, Millis S, McKinley W, Tulsky D. Late neurologic recovery after traumatic spinal cord injury. Arch Phys Med Rehabil 2004; 85(11): 1811-7.
[http://dx.doi.org/10.1016/j.apmr.2004.03.015] [PMID: 15520976]

[52]   Chernykh ER, Stupak VV, Muradov GM, *et al.* Application of autologous bone marrow stem cells in the therapy of spinal cord injury patients. Bull Exp Biol Med 2007; 143(4): 543-7.
[http://dx.doi.org/10.1007/s10517-007-0175-y] [PMID: 18214319]

[53]   Dai G, Liu X, Zhang Z, Yang Z, Dai Y, Xu R. Transplantation of autologous bone marrow mesenchymal stem cells in the treatment of complete and chronic cervical spinal cord injury. Brain Res 2013; 1533: 73-9.
[http://dx.doi.org/10.1016/j.brainres.2013.08.016] [PMID: 23948102]

[54]   Jiang PC, Xiong WP, Wang G, *et al.* A clinical trial report of autologous bone marrow-derived mesenchymal stem cell transplantation in patients with spinal cord injury. Exp Ther Med 2013; 6(1): 140-6.
[http://dx.doi.org/10.3892/etm.2013.1083] [PMID: 23935735]

[55]   Karamouzian S, Nematollahi-Mahani SN, Nakhaee N, Eskandary H. Clinical safety and primary efficacy of bone marrow mesenchymal cell transplantation in subacute spinal cord injured patients. Clin Neurol Neurosurg 2012; 114(7): 935-9.
[http://dx.doi.org/10.1016/j.clineuro.2012.02.003] [PMID: 22464434]

[56]   Park JH, Kim DY, Sung IY, *et al.* Long-term results of spinal cord injury therapy using mesenchymal stem cells derived from bone marrow in humans. Neurosurgery 2012; 70(5): 1238-47.
[http://dx.doi.org/10.1227/NEU.0b013e31824387f9] [PMID: 22127044]

[57]   Watanabe S, Uchida K, Nakajima H, *et al.* Early transplantation of mesenchymal stem cells after spinal cord injury relieves pain hypersensitivity through suppression of pain-related signaling cascades and reduced inflammatory cell recruitment. Stem Cells 2015; 33(6): 1902-14.
[http://dx.doi.org/10.1002/stem.2006] [PMID: 25809552]

CHAPTER 10

Uses in Spine Surgery

Asser A. Sallam[1,*], Amr Sami Hussien[2] and **Oscar Garcia Casas[3]**

[1] *Department of Trauma and Orthopedic Surgery, Suez Canal University Hospitals, Ismailia, Egypt*

[2] *Warwick University Hospital, Warwick, UK*

[3] *Ashford and St Peter's NHS Trust, Chertsey, UK*

Abstract: The use of autogenous bone marrow aspirate concentrate (BMAC) may offer a nonsurgical treatment of lumbar degenerative disc disease. It can also be used to enhance the cervical spine fusion. This chapter focuses on: the feasibility for using BMAC in spine surgery, host factors that may affect the outcome, the local morbidity of aspiration, and outcome after application of BMAC.

Keywords: Bone Marrow, Bone Marrow Aspirate Concentrate (BMAC), Spinal surgery, Stem Cells.

INTRODUCTION

Moderate to severe symptomatic lumbar degenerative disc disease can be treated either by conservative therapy or fusion. The utilization of autogenous bone marrow aspirate concentrate (BMAC) may offer a nonsurgical treatment for this disease or it may be used to enhance cervical or lumbar spine fusion. We aim to assess the feasibility for using BMAC in spine surgery, analyze host factors that may affect the outcome and the local morbidity of aspiration.

CONSERVATIVE THERAPY FOR CERVICAL AND LUMBAR DEGENERATIVE DISC DISEASE

Degenerative disc disease (DDD) is defined as a progressive damage of intervertebral discs leading to pain and loss of disc height; the exact cause of disc degeneration is unclear. There is still controversy in correlation between disc degeneration and biomechanical stresses [1 - 3]. At a cellular level, nutrients spread through the capillary network in the vertebral body, then diffuse through

---

* **Corresponding author Asser A. Sallam:** Department of Trauma and Orthopedic Surgery, Suez Canal University Hospitals, Ismailia, Egypt; Tel: +20 109 52772120; E-mail: assersallam@hotmail.com

Mohamed A Imam and Martyn Snow (Eds.)

the endplate into the extracellular matrix of the disc to reach the nucleus pulposus [4].

Endplates calcification ameliorates the flow of the nutrients *e.g.* glucose and oxygen [5]. It also aggravates the hypoxic acidic medium further damaging the disc cell metabolism [6].

Production of pro-inflammatory molecules (such as TNF-α and interleukins) as well as an intensification of local acidity were caused by repeated stresses, acute trauma, or natural disc degeneration. The collective influences of inflammatory environments and nutrient lack lead to a reduction in proteoglycan synthesis and consequently death of nucleus pulposus cell [7, 8].

Recently, bone marrows aspirate concentrate (BMAC) has been proposed for utilization in regenerative medicine [9, 10]. BMAC contains various stem and progenitor cells, including mesenchymal stem cells (MSCs). Various experimental studies documented the anti-inflammatory properties of MSCs in osteoarthritis, renal ischemia and reperfusion injury, myocardial infarction, hepatic cell failure, burns and autoimmune encephalomyelitis [11 - 17].

Some studies performed *in vitro* suggest that the regenerative capacity of MSCs may be attributed to the interaction between the nucleus pulposus cells and MSCs in managing disc degeneration. For example, Sobajima *et al.* reported that culturing the bone marrow-derived MSCs together with nucleus pulposus cells had a synergistic effect on increasing the proteoglycan synthesis and glycosaminoglycan content [18].

There are some reports on the safety of utilizing autogenous BMAC in treatment of moderate to severe lumbar DDD. The first was published by Pettine in 2014 [19]; 60 ml of bone marrow aspirate were obtained through percutaneous aspiration of the posterior iliac wing and were then concentrated. Then, they injected 2-3 ml of BMAC into each symptomatic lumbar nucleus pulposus using a two-needle discography method. They reported no complications and suggested that autogenous BMAC may be beneficial in treating DDD conservatively.

Another study published by Pettine *et al.* in 2015 [20] emphasized the safety and feasibility of using BMAC in the conservative treatment of pain arising from DDD. Twenty-six patients (median age: 40 (18-61) years) received autologous BMAC disc injections (13 one level and 13 two levels). Nearly, one ml of BMAC was analyzed for colony-forming unit-fibroblast (CFU-F) frequency, total nucleated cell (TNC) content, potential of differentiation, and phenotyping. Using fluoroscopy, the BMAC was injected into the symptomatic disc nucleus. The average pain and disability scores were reduced during one-year follow-up period.

About 121×10^6 TNC/ml with 2,713 CFU-F/ml (synonymous with mesenchymal stem cells) were counted in the average BMAC. Although there is a considerable pain reduction in all patients, patients receiving greater than 2,000 CFU-F/ml developed a significantly faster and greater reduction in discogenic pain and functional disability. The authors followed-up the patients for another year and concluded that BMAC could be considered an alternative procedure for spine surgery, with durable pain relief (71% Visual Analog Scale reduction) and Oswestry Disability Index improvements (> 64%) through two years [21].

BONE GRAFTING FOR SPINAL FUSION

Tricortical iliac crest is traditionally used for bone grafting in anterior cervical fusion. Up till now, graft harvesting can lead to donor site morbidity, limited graft volume and limited re-harvesting possibility. Bone Marrow Aspiration (BMA) is less invasive and offers a rich source of regenerative cells. Enrichment of BMA can be performed, forming a bone marrow aspirate concentrate (BMAC) that can be added to allografts.

The quality of BMAC obtained from the anterior iliac crest to be utilized in cervical fusion, patient factors that may affect the quality of the aspirate, or the donor morbidity have not yet well-investigated. Gregory *et al.* [22] suggested that BMAC might provide osteoprogenitor cells to the fusion site with minimal donor site morbidity. Tobacco use and age are negatively affecting the numbers of CFU.

In relation to donor site morbidity following aspiration from the iliac crest, Chaput *et al.* [23] recorded minimal to no pain using VAS at 3-6 months post-harvest. The CFU-F frequency in bone marrow equals or exceeds literature-reported values, with more than 40% of the CFUs representing cells with osteogenic potential; greater than a 3-fold enrichment was demonstrated for both CFU-F and CFU-O on average. These findings suggest that there is BMAC can provide osteoprogenitor cells to the fusion site with little or no donor site morbidity.

Vadala *et al.* [24] described a case of s multi-diseased osteoporotic patient affected by cervical canal stenosis, aged 88 years. This patient underwent a C3-C7 posterior decompression, instrumentation and posterolateral fusion; using a corticocancellous bone allograft imprignated with autologous BMAC enriched with platelet-rich fibrin (PRF). At 6 months postoperatively, X-rays and CT scan showed solid C3-C7 fusion. However, a recent study [25] concluded that there was no statistical difference between autologous BMAC mixed with allograft cancellous bone and iliac crest autograft regarding fusion scores in lumbar region.

SUMMARY

The use of BMAC and expanded stem cells demonstrate promising initial results and could be used, in the future, in managing various spinal problems.

CONSENT FOR PUBLICATION

Not applicable.

CONFLICT OF INTEREST

The authors declare no conflict of interest, financial or otherwise.

ACKNOWLEDGEMENTS

Declared none.

REFERENCES

[1]   Ching CT, Chow DH, Yao FY, Holmes AD. The effect of cyclic compression on the mechanical properties of the inter-vertebral disc: an *in vivo* study in a rat tail model. Clin Biomech (Bristol, Avon) 2003; 18(3): 182-9.
        [http://dx.doi.org/10.1016/S0268-0033(02)00188-2] [PMID: 12620780]

[2]   Kroeber MW, Unglaub F, Wang H, *et al.* New *in vivo* animal model to create intervertebral disc degeneration and to investigate the effects of therapeutic strategies to stimulate disc regeneration. Spine 2002; 27(23): 2684-90.
        [http://dx.doi.org/10.1097/00007632-200212010-00007] [PMID: 12461394]

[3]   Yamazaki S, Weinhold PS, Graff RD, *et al.* Annulus cells release ATP in response to vibratory loading *in vitro*. J Cell Biochem 2003; 90(4): 812-8.
        [http://dx.doi.org/10.1002/jcb.10681] [PMID: 14587036]

[4]   Frymoyer JW, Gordon SL. American Academy of Orthopaedic Surgeons. New perspectives on low back pain : workshop, Airlie, Virginia, May 1988. Park Ridge, Ill., The Academy.

[5]   Roberts S, Menage J, Eisenstein SM. The cartilage end-plate and intervertebral disc in scoliosis: calcification and other sequelae. J Orthop Res 1993; 11(5): 747-57.
        [http://dx.doi.org/10.1002/jor.1100110517] [PMID: 8410475]

[6]   Bartels EM, Fairbank JC, Winlove CP, Urban JP. Oxygen and lactate concentrations measured *in vivo* in the intervertebral discs of patients with scoliosis and back pain. Spine 1998; 23(1): 1-7.
        [http://dx.doi.org/10.1097/00007632-199801010-00001] [PMID: 9460145]

[7]   Bibby SR, Urban JP. Effect of nutrient deprivation on the viability of intervertebral disc cells. Eur Spine J 2004; 13(8): 695-701.
        [http://dx.doi.org/10.1007/s00586-003-0616-x] [PMID: 15048560]

[8]   Horner HA, Urban JP. 2001 Volvo Award Winner in Basic Science Studies: Effect of nutrient supply on the viability of cells from the nucleus pulposus of the intervertebral disc. Spine 2001; 26(23): 2543-9.
        [http://dx.doi.org/10.1097/00007632-200112010-00006] [PMID: 11725234]

[9]   Murphy MB, Blashki D, Buchanan RM, *et al.* Adult and umbilical cord blood-derived platelet-rich plasma for mesenchymal stem cell proliferation, chemotaxis, and cryo-preservation. Biomaterials 2012; 33(21): 5308-16.

[http://dx.doi.org/10.1016/j.biomaterials.2012.04.007] [PMID: 22542609]

[10]   Moncivais K, Caplan AI. Mesenchymal stem cells: environmentally responsive therapeutics for regenerative medicine. E Exp Mol Med 2013; 45: e54.
[http://dx.doi.org/10.1038/emm.2013.94]

[11]   Black LL, Gaynor J, Gahring D, *et al.* Effect of adipose-derived mesenchymal stem and regenerative cells on lameness in dogs with chronic osteoarthritis of the coxofemoral joints: a randomized, double-blinded, multicenter, controlled trial. Vet Ther 2007; 8(4): 272-84.
[PMID: 18183546]

[12]   Black LL, Gaynor J, Adams C, *et al.* Effect of intraarticular injection of autologous adipose-derived mesenchymal stem and regenerative cells on clinical signs of chronic osteoarthritis of the elbow joint in dogs. Vet Ther 2008; 9(3): 192-200.
[PMID: 19003780]

[13]   Ohnishi S, Yanagawa B, Tanaka K, *et al.* Transplantation of mesenchymal stem cells attenuates myocardial injury and dysfunction in a rat model of acute myocarditis. J Mol Cell Cardiol 2007; 42(1): 88-97.
[http://dx.doi.org/10.1016/j.yjmcc.2006.10.003] [PMID: 17101147]

[14]   Semedo P, Wang PM, Andreucci TH, *et al.* Mesenchymal stem cells ameliorate tissue damages triggered by renal ischemia and reperfusion injury. Transplant Proc 2007; 39(2): 421-3.
[http://dx.doi.org/10.1016/j.transproceed.2007.01.036] [PMID: 17362746]

[15]   Parekkadan B, van Poll D, Suganuma K, *et al.* Mesenchymal stem cell-derived molecules reverse fulminant hepatic failure. PLoS One 2007; 2(9): e941.
[http://dx.doi.org/10.1371/journal.pone.0000941] [PMID: 17895982]

[16]   Gerdoni E, Gallo B, Casazza S, *et al.* Mesenchymal stem cells effectively modulate pathogenic immune response in experimental autoimmune encephalomyelitis. Ann Neurol 2007; 61(3): 219-27.
[http://dx.doi.org/10.1002/ana.21076] [PMID: 17387730]

[17]   Rasulov MF, Vasilenko VT, Zaidenov VA, Onishchenko NA. Cell transplantation inhibits inflammatory reaction and stimulates repair processes in burn wound. Bull Exp Biol Med 2006; 142(1): 112-5.
[http://dx.doi.org/10.1007/s10517-006-0306-x] [PMID: 17369918]

[18]   Sobajima S, Vadala G, Shimer A, Kim JS, Gilbertson LG, Kang JD. Feasibility of a stem cell therapy for intervertebral disc degeneration. Spine J 2008; 8(6): 888-96.
[http://dx.doi.org/10.1016/j.spinee.2007.09.011] [PMID: 18082460]

[19]   Pettine KA. Autogenous Point of Care Bone Marrow Concentrate (BMC) for the Treatment of Lumbar Degenerative Disc Disease: IRB Controlled Prospective Study. Spine J 2014; 14(11): S30-1.
[http://dx.doi.org/10.1016/j.spinee.2014.08.082]

[20]   Pettine KA, Murphy MB, Suzuki RK, Sand TT. Percutaneous injection of autologous bone marrow concentrate cells significantly reduces lumbar discogenic pain through 12 months. Stem Cells 2015; 33(1): 146-56.
[http://dx.doi.org/10.1002/stem.1845] [PMID: 25187512]

[21]   Pettine K, Suzuki R, Sand T, Murphy M. Treatment of discogenic back pain with autologous bone marrow concentrate injection with minimum two year follow-up. Int Orthop 2016; 40(1): 135-40.
[http://dx.doi.org/10.1007/s00264-015-2886-4] [PMID: 26156727]

[22]   Gregory C, Chaput CD, Clough B. Bone Marrow Aspirate Quality from the Anterior Iliac Crest in Relationship to Age, Gender and Tobacco Use. Spine J 2012; 12(9): S58.
[http://dx.doi.org/10.1016/j.spinee.2012.08.163]

[23]   Chaput C, Zeitouni S, Clough B, Sampson W. Donor site morbidity and in vitro analysis of the osteogenic potential of bone marrow aspirate concentrate from the anterior iliac crest. Spine J 2011; 11(10): S59.

[http://dx.doi.org/10.1016/j.spinee.2011.08.150]

[24]   Vadalà G, Di Martino A, Tirindelli MC, Denaro L, Denaro V. Use of autologous bone marrow cells concentrate enriched with platelet-rich fibrin on corticocancellous bone allograft for posterolateral multilevel cervical fusion. J Tissue Eng Regen Med 2008; 2(8): 515-20.
[http://dx.doi.org/10.1002/term.121] [PMID: 18972577]

[25]   Johnson RG. Bone marrow concentrate with allograft equivalent to autograft in lumbar fusions. S Spine (Phila Pa 1976) 2014 Apr 20;39(9):695-700.

CHAPTER 11

Role of BMAC in Tendinitis or Tendon Pathology

Saman Horriat[1,*], Mohamed A. Imam[2], Lukas Ernstbrunner[3] and **Rohit Gupta[4]**

[1] *St George's Hospital, London, UK*

[2] *The Royal Orthopaedic Hospital, Birmingham, B31 2AP, UK; Suez Canal University Hospitals, Ismailia, 41111, Egypt*

[3] *Department of Orthopaedics, Balgrist University Hospital, University of Zurich, Forchstrasse 340, 8008 Zurich, Switzerland; Department of Orthopaedics and Traumatology Paracelsus Medical University, Muellner Hauptstrasse 48, 5020, Salzburg, Austria*

[4] *Ashford and St Peter's NHS hospital, Surrey, UK*

Abstract: Tendon pathologies represent a group of musculoskeletal conditions commonly viewed in orthopaedic and rheumatology clinics. They are classified into traumatic, degenerative and over-use related types. As yet, the majority of conventional approaches have unpredictable results and regularly fail to produce satisfying clinical recovery. With increasing indication of the successful utilisation of MSCs in different divisions of medicine, there is significant interest in employing expanded stem cells to manage these pathologies. Here, we investigate written reports concerning the employment of MSC for managing tendon pathologies.

Keywords: Bone Marrow, Bone Marrow Aspirate Concentrate (BMAC), Stem Cells, Tendon pathology.

INTRODUCTION

Till lately, it was broadly accepted that after the application of MSCs, the cells change into the target cells and engage in the repair process. Notwithstanding, new studies proposed that healing potential of MSCs are essentially through chemical cytokines which can interact with the damaged tissue and guide cell proliferation, angiogenesis and inflammatory processes needed for reconstruction [1 - 7].

Unluckily, there are quite limited reported studies on the influence of MSC on tendons regeneration, yet, the current evidence is summarised in this chapter.

---

[*] **Corresponding author Saman Horriat:** St George's Hospital, London, UK; E-mail: SamanHorriat@gmail.com

Mohamed A Imam and Martyn Snow (Eds.)

SELECTED EVIDENCE FROM LABORATORY AND PRE-CLINICAL STUDIES

Gulotta *et al.* (2009, 2010, 2011), in a series of studies, claim that MSC alone did not have a significant effect on healing or the biomechanical properties of rotator cuff repair in an animal model. Nonetheless, augmented MSC either with Scleraxis (helix transcription factor) or with MT1-MMP (membrane type 1 matrix metalloproteinase): a developmental gene, could improve rotator cuff healing, increase biomechanical strength and reduce re-rupture in rats [8 - 11].

Kim *et al.* (2013) showed the survival of labelled MSCs in tendon repair and also increased a concentration of collagen type I in rabbits' rotator cuff repair in the presence of MSCs [12]. Zhao *et al.* (2009), in their *ex-vivo study*, tested the maximal strength of repaired canine FDP tendons in the presence of harvested bone marrow stromal cells and demonstrated stronger repair at four weeks in the study group (using stem cell-seeded gel patch) [13].

Renzi *et al.* (2013) examined autologous MSC when used in managing tendinitis on racehorses as an animal model for high-performance athletes. In this study, the concentrate of marrow aspirate from the sternum of racehorses enhanced the function of 13/18 horses and enabled them to revert back to competitive levels [14].

Furthermore, Torricelli *et al.* (2011), in a different small preclinical series, on Racehorses, used MSCs and Platelet Rich Plasma (PRP) to manage tendon and ligament injuries. They published significant improvement in all animals and a return to racing in 84% of the horses [15].

Godwin *et al.* (2011), in the largest non-human case series on the effect of MSC injection on tendon injuries, reported over 98% return to racing in 113 race-horses with superficial digital flexor tendon injury treated with an ultrasound-guided injection of MSC [16]. Finally, Smith *et al.* (2013), in another preclinical study analysed at histological, molecular and biomechanical characteristics of injured tendons of racehorses treated with MSCs. In their study, 12 horses with superficial digital flexor tendon injuries were randomised into the treatment group with MSC and control group which received an injection of saline. Following a six months rehabilitation programme, tendons of all horses tested for vascularity, cellularity, water content, DNA content, GAG and MMP-13 content. They also tested for crimp pattern, elasticity modulus and structural stiffness. According to their study results, the authors concluded that injured tendons treated with MSC showed biochemical, histological and biomechanical characteristics similar to the normal tendon compared with the control group [17].

CLINICAL EVIDENCE

Elbow Epicondylitis

Moon *et al.* (2008) published one of the first clinical studies on BMAC uses in tendinopathies [18]. They coupled operative treatment with BMAC to treat epicondylitis in 26 elbows (24 patients) which had failed non-operative treatment. Their approach included arthroscopic debridement and re-insertion of the affected tendons (common flexor origin in golfers' elbow or ECRB in tennis elbow) and injection of 8 - 9 ml of buffy coat layer of BMA centrifuged for 15 minutes at 1800 rpm. Patients started their rehabilitation programme after 2 days of immobilization in a splint. They assessed clinical outcomes using VAS pain score and Mayo Elbow Performance (MEP) score, which showed significant improvement in their final follow up at six months compared to their baseline scores.

Singh *et al.* (2014) reported clinical outcomes of local injection of BMAC for patients with lateral epicondylitis (tennis elbow) based on PRTEE (Patient-Rated Tennis Elbow Evaluation) score. They recruited a group of 30 patients (18 male and 12 female) with a clinical diagnosis of tennis elbow aged between 18 and 65. Their patients received a single injection of 4-5 ml of buffy coat layer from 10 ml autologous BMA centrifuged for 20 minutes at 2000 rpm. At 12 weeks, there was a significant increase in average PRTEE score in comparison with the initial score (72.8 +/- 6.9 down to 14.86 +/- 3.48). The authors concluded that the application of growth factors including regenerative cells in BMAC was an efficient strategy to manage chronic tendinopathy [19].

ROTATOR CUFF TEARS

Various studies assessed the purported advantage of using BMAC in augmenting repairs of the rotator cuff tendons (Table **1**). Heringou *et al.* (2014), in their study, investigated the integrity of single row rotator cuff repair augmented with BMAC in a group of 45 patients. They followed the patients up using ultrasound and MRI scans at 3, 6, 12 and 24 months and at final follow up at ten years. Their results compared with a matched control group of 45 patients who only had rotator cuff repair without biologic augmentation.

They report 100% healed repair at 6 months in the study group compared with 67% in control group; with a re-rupture rate of 13% in the study group compared to 56% in the control group. Finally, the authors concluded that using BMAC as a biological augment for rotator cuff repair can significantly improve healing outcome of tendon repair and long-term integrity of the repaired tendon [20].

Table 1. Summary of uses of BMAC in rotator cuff pathology.

Study ID	Design	Population	Intervention	Comparator	Outcome measure	Findings
Gomes *et al.*	Single arm prospective study	Fourteen patients (9 women, 5 men) with full thickness rotator cuff tears	Trans-osseous stitches augmented with BMAC utilising a mini open technique.	No control	University of California Los Angeles	from 12 ± 3.0 to 31 ± 3.2
					Tendon integrity (12 months)	Tendon integrity was maintained in 100% of cases.
Hernigou *et al.*	Prospective, matched-control, study	fifty-four patients	BMAC in augmenting arthroscopic single row rotator cuff repair	Matched control group of forty-five patients without augmentation with BMAC	Tendon integrity (6 months)	100% *vs.* 67%
					Tendon integrity (10 years)	87% *vs.* 44%
Centeno *et al.*	Prospective multicentre cohort study	Patients with osteoarthritis with and without rotator cuff pathology	BMAC injection for the glenohumeral OA	None	-The arm, shoulder and hand score -Visual analogue score - Mean subjective improvement	- Improved from 36.1 to 17.1 (P<0.001) - Improved from 4.3 to 2.4 (P<0.001) - 48.8%

Gomes *et al.* (2011) investigated clinical and radiological outcomes of added BMAC to the conventional mini-open rotator cuff repair using UCLA score and MRI scan at 12 months follow up. In their study, 14 patients were repaired using trans-osseous stitches augmented with an injection of BMAC at the Tendon-Bone interface. They reported significant UCLA score improvement at 12 months; superior tendon integration on MRI scan at 12 months [21].

Similarly, Havlas *et al.* (2015) in case series of 8 patients, who received cultivated bone marrow stem cells at the suture sites, after arthroscopic rotator cuff repair reported excellent outcome compared to their pre-operative condition. In their study, VAS pain score was 0 at six months, with significant improvement in both UCLA and Constant score both at 3 and 6 months postoperatively. MRI scan at the final follow-up demonstrated entirely healed and integrated repair. In their definitive conclusion, they advocated additional studies and claimed that the application of concentrated marrow stem cells is safe and effective when used to augment rotator cuff repair [22].

PATELLA TENDINITS

Pascual-Garrido *et al.* (2012), in a case series, published superior patient satisfaction and improved clinical outcomes when they have employed BMAC to manage refractory patella tendinitis that was unresponsive to conservative therapy. They reported the clinical outcomes in 8 patients, aged between 14 and 35 years. They have observed significant improvement in pain and enhanced return to activity of daily living as evident by the significant increase in knee-related quality of life and functional knee scores (IKDC and KOOS) in 7 patients. Those seven patients would have the procedure again and all seven graded their final outcome as excellent [23].

ACHILLES TENDON

Stein *et al.* (2015), studied 27 patients (28 tendons) presenting with Achilles tendon rupture, all sustained in athletes. All patients were managed with open tendon repair that was augmented with the injection of BMAC. They reported excellent improved functional results with insignificant complications. At an average of two and a half years post-surgery, there was no retears and the mean Achilles tendon Total Rupture Score was 91 (best equaling 100). They described a return to full sporting activities at six months in 25 of 27 patients. they reported one superficial wound dehiscence which presented the most significant complication, without any occurrence of infection or other medical complications (DVT/PE) [24].

CONCLUSION

We have investigated the clinical uses of BMAC to manage tendon pathologies using the available literature. Unfortunately, as yet, there is scarcely available proof both in terms of the level of evidence and the number of published studies. The published articles do not publish a vital complication that is directly related to the application of BMAC when used in tendon pathologies; yet, apart from one study with a ten year follow up [20], all additional clinical studies had short or medium term follow up.

SUMMARY

In our view, while the current evidence explicates encouraging outcomes for managing tendinopathy and enhancing repair, BMAC is not highly recommended in tendon pathologies. This is essentially due to the insufficient quantity and quality of studies, which are principally retrospective case series. There is a need for further well designed clinical studies in the subject.

CONSENT FOR PUBLICATION

Not applicable.

CONFLICT OF INTEREST

The authors declare no conflict of interest, financial or otherwise.

ACKNOWLEDGEMENTS

Declared none.

REFERENCES

[1]   Pereira RF, Halford KW, O'Hara MD, *et al.* Cultured adherent cells from marrow can serve as long-lasting precursor cells for bone, cartilage, and lung in irradiated mice. Proc Natl Acad Sci USA 1995; 92(11): 4857-61.
        [http://dx.doi.org/10.1073/pnas.92.11.4857] [PMID: 7761413]

[2]   Pereira RF, O'Hara MD, Laptev AV, *et al.* Marrow stromal cells as a source of progenitor cells for nonhematopoietic tissues in transgenic mice with a phenotype of osteogenesis imperfecta. Proc Natl Acad Sci USA 1998; 95(3): 1142-7.
        [http://dx.doi.org/10.1073/pnas.95.3.1142] [PMID: 9448299]

[3]   Chopp M, Li Y, Zhang ZG. Mechanisms underlying improved recovery of neurological function after stroke in the rodent after treatment with neurorestorative cell-based therapies. Stroke 2009; 40(3) (Suppl.): S143-5.
        [http://dx.doi.org/10.1161/STROKEAHA.108.533141] [PMID: 19064763]

[4]   Tögel F, Westenfelder C. The role of multipotent marrow stromal cells (MSCs) in tissue regeneration. Organogenesis 2011; 7(2): 96-100.
        [http://dx.doi.org/10.4161/org.7.2.15781] [PMID: 21521944]

[5]   Schwarz SC, Schwarz J. Translation of stem cell therapy for neurological diseases. Transl Res 2010; 156(3): 155-60.
        [http://dx.doi.org/10.1016/j.trsl.2010.07.002] [PMID: 20801412]

[6]   Alaiti MA, Ishikawa M, Costa MA. Bone marrow and circulating stem/progenitor cells for regenerative cardiovascular therapy. Transl Res 2010; 156(3): 112-29.
        [http://dx.doi.org/10.1016/j.trsl.2010.06.008] [PMID: 20801408]

[7]   Fernández Vallone VB, Romaniuk MA, Choi H, Labovsky V, Otaegui J, Chasseing NA. Mesenchymal stem cells and their use in therapy: what has been achieved? Differentiation 2013; 85(1-2): 1-10.
        [http://dx.doi.org/10.1016/j.diff.2012.08.004] [PMID: 23314286]

[8]   Gulotta LV, Kovacevic D, Ehteshami JR, Dagher E, Packer JD, Rodeo SA. Application of bone marrow-derived mesenchymal stem cells in a rotator cuff repair model. Am J Sports Med 2009; 37(11): 2126-33.
        [http://dx.doi.org/10.1177/0363546509339582] [PMID: 19684297]

[9]   Gulotta LV, Kovacevic D, Montgomery S, Ehteshami JR, Packer JD, Rodeo SA. Stem cells genetically modified with the developmental gene MT1-MMP improve regeneration of the supraspinatus tendon-to-bone insertion site. Am J Sports Med 2010; 38(7): 1429-37.
        [http://dx.doi.org/10.1177/0363546510361235] [PMID: 20400753]

[10] Gulotta LV, Kovacevic D, Packer JD, Deng XH, Rodeo SA. Bone marrow-derived mesenchymal stem cells transduced with scleraxis improve rotator cuff healing in a rat model. Am J Sports Med 2011; 39(6): 1282-9.
[http://dx.doi.org/10.1177/0363546510395485] [PMID: 21335341]

[11] Gulotta LV, Kovacevic D, Packer JD, Ehteshami JR, Rodeo SA. Adenoviral-mediated gene transfer of human bone morphogenetic protein-13 does not improve rotator cuff healing in a rat model. Am J Sports Med 2011; 39(1): 180-7.
[http://dx.doi.org/10.1177/0363546510379339] [PMID: 20956264]

[12] Kim YS, Bigliani LU, Fujisawa M, *et al.* Stromal cell-derived factor 1 (SDF-1, CXCL12) is increased in subacromial bursitis and downregulated by steroid and nonsteroidal anti-inflammatory agents. J Orthop Res 2006; 24(8): 1756-64.
[http://dx.doi.org/10.1002/jor.20197] [PMID: 16779827]

[13] Zhao C, Chieh HF, Bakri K, *et al.* The effects of bone marrow stromal cell transplants on tendon healing *in vitro.* Med Eng Phys 2009; 31(10): 1271-5.
[http://dx.doi.org/10.1016/j.medengphy.2009.08.004] [PMID: 19736035]

[14] Renzi S, Riccò S, Dotti S, *et al.* Autologous bone marrow mesenchymal stromal cells for regeneration of injured equine ligaments and tendons: a clinical report. Res Vet Sci 2013; 95(1): 272-7.
[http://dx.doi.org/10.1016/j.rvsc.2013.01.017] [PMID: 23419936]

[15] Torricelli P, Fini M, Filardo G, *et al.* Regenerative medicine for the treatment of musculoskeletal overuse injuries in competition horses Int orth 2011; 35(10): 1569-1576
[http://dx.doi.org/10.1007/s00264-011-1237-3]

[16] Godwin EE, Young NJ, Dudhia J, Beamish IC, Smith RK. Implantation of bone marrow-derived mesenchymal stem cells demonstrates improved outcome in horses with overstrain injury of the superficial digital flexor tendon. Equine Vet J 2012; 44(1): 25-32.
[http://dx.doi.org/10.1111/j.2042-3306.2011.00363.x] [PMID: 21615465]

[17] Smith RK, Werling NJ, Dakin SG, Alam R, Goodship AE, Dudhia J. Beneficial effects of autologous bone marrow-derived mesenchymal stem cells in naturally occurring tendinopathy. PLoS One 2013; 8(9): e75697.
[http://dx.doi.org/10.1371/journal.pone.0075697] [PMID: 24086616]

[18] Moon YL, Jo SH, Song CH, Park G, Lee HJ, Jang SJ. Autologous bone marrow plasma injection after arthroscopic debridement for elbow tendinosis. Ann Acad Med Singapore 2008; 37(7): 559-63.
[PMID: 18695767]

[19] Singh A, Gangwar DS, Singh S. Bone marrow injection: A novel treatment for tennis elbow. J Nat Sci Biol Med 2014; 5(2): 389-91.
[http://dx.doi.org/10.4103/0976-9668.136198] [PMID: 25097421]

[20] Hernigou P, Flouzat Lachaniette CH, Delambre J, *et al.* Biologic augmentation of rotator cuff repair with mesenchymal stem cells during arthroscopy improves healing and prevents further tears: a case-controlled study. Int Orthop 2014; 38(9): 1811-8.
[http://dx.doi.org/10.1007/s00264-014-2391-1] [PMID: 24913770]

[21] Ellera Gomes JL, da Silva RC, Silla LM, Abreu MR, Pellanda R. Conventional rotator cuff repair complemented by the aid of mononuclear autologous stem cells. Knee Surg Sports Traumatol Arthrosc 2012; 20(2): 373-7.
[http://dx.doi.org/10.1007/s00167-011-1607-9] [PMID: 21773831]

[22] Havlas V, Kotaška J, Koníček P, *et al.* [Use of cultured human autologous bone marrow stem cells in repair of a rotator cuff tear: preliminary results of a safety study]. Acta Chir Orthop Traumatol Cech 2015; 82(3): 229-34. [Czech.].
[PMID: 26317295]

[23]   Pascual-Garrido C, Rolón A, Makino A. Treatment of chronic patellar tendinopathy with autologous bone marrow stem cells: a 5-year-followup. Stem Cells Int 2012; 2012: 953510.
[http://dx.doi.org/10.1155/2012/953510] [PMID: 22220180]

[24]   Stein BE, Stroh DA, Schon LC. Outcomes of acute Achilles tendon rupture repair with bone marrow aspirate concentrate augmentation. Int Orthop 2015; 39(5): 901-5.
[http://dx.doi.org/10.1007/s00264-015-2725-7] [PMID: 25795246]

CHAPTER 12

BMAC in Foot and Ankle Surgery

Mohamed A. Imam[1,2,*], **Mohamed Shehata**[3], **Saqib Javed**[2] and **Arshad Khaleel**[5]

[1] *The Royal Orthopaedic Hospital, Birmingham, B31 2AP, UK*

[2] *Wrightington Hospital, Appley Bridge, Wigan, UK*

[3] *Faculty of Medicine, Zagazig University, 44741, Egypt*

[4] *Ashford and St Peter's NHS Trust, UK*

Abstract: In this chapter, we aim to describe the current literature published on the uses of BMAC in the management of foot and ankle disorders. Animal and human studies suggest promising results on the usage of BMAC in augmenting arthrodesis and bone healing. Little evidence is published demonstrating the potential benefits of BMAC used in conjunction with foot and ankle surgery.

Keywords: Bone Marrow, Bone Marrow Aspirate Concentrate (BMAC), Charcot arthropathy, Foot and ankle surgery, Stem Cells.

INTRODUCTION

Arthrodesis remains the mainstay of treatment for advanced stages of arthritis of the joints of the foot and ankle. Patients who smoke or suffer from diabetes are at an increased risk of developing complications such as nonunion and this can be as high as 40% leading to persistent pain and debilitation [1 - 5]; alternative methods of achieving union in fusions are consequently being considered. Bone Marrow Aspirate Concentrate (BMAC) has been successfully used for bone and soft-tissue healing [6, 7]. The purported advantage is the harvest and administration of viable cells and growth factors. BMAC contains multipotent stem cells (MSCs), hematopoietic stem cells (HSCs), endothelial progenitor cells and other progenitor cells, as well as growth factors, including bone morphogenetic proteins [6, 7].

Although BMA comprises similar components, the additional concentration of BMA usually leads to improved healing. This is mainly because of a theoretical critical number of certain cellular components and which is not related to the entire cell count [8].

* **Corresponding author Mohamed A. Imam:** The Royal Orthopaedic Hospital, Birmingham, B31 2AP, UK; Tel; +44 121 685 4000; Fax: +44 121 685 4100; E-mail: Mohamed.Imam@aol.com

Furthermore, in foot and ankle surgery there is limited physical space for implantation of biologics. Consequently, BMAC is an attractive solution to overcome this difficulty. Both the MSCs and HSCs have the potential to differentiate into osteogenic progenitors. This differentiation can happen with the help of growth factors and induction proteins, either locally where the BMAC is administered, or by the elements contained in the BMAC. Additionally, the cells contained within the BMAC have a paracrine effect on attract extra cells to the location and enhance additional growth factor protein production in a paracrine fashion. Although, there are hypothetical benefits of BMAC, no long-term level-one evidence for BMAC use is available currently. In this chapter, we aim to review the foot and ankle literature for the use of BMAC.

ANIMAL EVIDENCE

Several animal studies demonstrated the use of BMAC in bone healing. In 2016, Gianakos *et al*. [9] undertook a review assessing the available evidence published on the uses of BMAC in long-bone healing in animals. They reported significant encouraging evidence for BMAC use. Of the studies reporting statistics on the outcomes of the usage of BMAC, 100% showed a significant increase in bone formation in the BMAC groups compared with controls. Moreover, radiological studies have shown a significant increase in the production of both callus volume and woven bone. With subsequent higher rates of union achieved in the BMAC group compared with the control group. Histological analyses confirmed radiographic findings of significant improvement in osteocyte quantity and activity as well as bone formation.

Conversely, Jungbluth *et al*. [10], demonstrated BMAC to be less effective in the management of metaphyseal defects. They compared the use of autograft, BMAC and calcium phosphate in the management of metaphyseal bone healing in the tibias of mini-pigs. The BMAC group exhibited significantly more bone formation compared with the calcium phosphate group but the autograft group demonstrated significantly more bone formation than the BMAC group.

HUMAN STUDIES

Few studies have described the utilization of BMAC in foot and ankle surgery. Murawski *et al*. [11] undertook percutaneous screw fixation augmented with BMAC for the management of proximal fifth metatarsal fractures in 26 patients. At an average follow-up of 21 months, 24 of these patients achieved union without complication at a mean of 5 weeks after surgery. 1/26 patients achieved delayed union and one re-fractured. Generally, this cohort of patients experienced a significant improvement in their Foot and Ankle Outcome Score and both the physical and mental components of the 12-Item short form survey.

Likewise, O'Malley *et al.* [12] retrospectively analysed the charts of 10 professional basketball players with Jones fractures managed with open reduction and internal fixation augmented with BMAC. They reported a mean time interval to fracture healing of seven and half weeks. Recurrence of fracture occurred in three patients. However, there are limitations in these two studies [11, 12]. Unfortunately, both studies lacked a control group making the results less meaningful.

Hernigou *et al.* [13] undertook a retrospective case-control study on 172 diabetic patients with ankle fracture nonunion. They divided the cohort into two groups; 86 who received BMAC injection *versus* 86 matched diabetic patients who received Iliac crest Bone Graft (IBG) for the treatment of the ankle fracture nonunions. In this study, 70/86 patients (82%) treated with BMAC showed bone healing compared with only 53/86 (62%) diabetic patients who undertook IBG. Additionally, the risk of complications was higher for the IBG group when compared to the BMAC group.

Similarly, Adams *et al.* [14] described a technique in which BMAC is delivered through a percutaneous cannulated screw to manage non healed stress fractures occurring in the medial cuneiform. The screw cannula is covered with wax and BMAC was injected through the wax into the cannula. Post operative CT scans confirmed subsequent healing of the stress fracture.

SUMMARY

There appears to be promising results on the use of BMAC in foot and ankle surgery. Further research is still required, particularly clinical trials to confirm the safety and efficacy of BMAC when used in foot and ankle surgery.

CONSENT FOR PUBLICATION

Not applicable.

CONFLICT OF INTEREST

The authors declare no conflict of interest, financial or otherwise.

ACKNOWLEDGEMENTS

Declared none.

REFERENCES

[1]   Dhote R, Charde P, Bhongade M, Rao J. Stem cells cultured on beta tricalcium phosphate (β-TCP) in combination with recombinant human platelet-derived growth factor - BB (rh-PDGF-BB) for

the treatment of human infrabony defects. J Stem Cells 2015; 10(4): 243-54.

[2]   McGuire MK, Scheyer ET, Snyder MB. Evaluation of recession defects treated with coronally advanced flaps and either recombinant human platelet-derived growth factor-BB plus β-tricalcium phosphate or connective tissue: comparison of clinical parameters at 5 years. J Periodontol 2014; 85(10): 1361-70.
[http://dx.doi.org/10.1902/jop.2014.140006] [PMID: 24694077]

[3]   Gugala Z. On a quest to dethrone the long-reigning king: commentary on an article by Christopher W. DiGiovanni, MD, *et al.*: "Recombinant Human platelet-derived growth factor-BB and beta-tricalcium phosphate (rhPDGF-BB/β-TCP): an alternative to autogenous bone graft". J Bone Joint Surg Am 2013; 95(13): e95.
[http://dx.doi.org/10.2106/JBJS.M.00677] [PMID: 23824400]

[4]   DiGiovanni CW, Lin SS, Baumhauer JF, *et al.* Recombinant human platelet-derived growth factor-BB and beta-tricalcium phosphate (rhPDGF-BB/β-TCP): an alternative to autogenous bone graft. J Bone Joint Surg Am 2013; 95(13): 1184-92.

[5]   Irokawa D, Ota M, Yamamoto S, Shibukawa Y, Yamada S. Effect of β tricalcium phosphate particle size on recombinant human platelet-derived growth factor-BB-induced regeneration of periodontal tissue in dog. Dent Mater J 2010; 29(6): 721-30.
[http://dx.doi.org/10.4012/dmj.2010-033] [PMID: 21099164]

[6]   Imam MA, Mahmoud SSS, Holton J, Abouelmaati D, Elsherbini Y, Snow M. A systematic review of the concept and clinical applications of Bone Marrow Aspirate Concentrate in Orthopaedics. SICOT J 2017; 3: 17.
[http://dx.doi.org/10.1051/sicotj/2017007]

[7]   Holton J, Imam M, Ward J, Snow M. The basic science of bone marrow aspirate concentrate in chondral injuries. Orthop Rev (Pavia) 2016; 8(3): 6659.
[http://dx.doi.org/10.4081/or.2016.6659] [PMID: 27761221]

[8]   Hernigou P, Poignard A, Beaujean F, Rouard H. Percutaneous autologous bone-marrow grafting for nonunions. Influence of the number and concentration of progenitor cells. J Bone Joint Surg Am 2005; 87(7): 1430-7.

[9]   Gianakos A, Ni A, Zambrana L, Kennedy JG, Lane JM. Bone marrow aspirate concentrate in animal long bone healing: an analysis of basic science evidence. J Orthop Trauma 2016; 30(1): 1-9.
[http://dx.doi.org/10.1097/BOT.0000000000000453] [PMID: 26371620]

[10]   Jungbluth P, Hakimi AR, Grassmann JP, *et al.* The early phase influence of bone marrow concentrate on metaphyseal bone healing. Injury 2013; 44(10): 1285-94.
[http://dx.doi.org/10.1016/j.injury.2013.04.015] [PMID: 23684350]

[11]   Murawski CD, Kennedy JG. Percutaneous internal fixation of proximal fifth metatarsal jones fractures (Zones II and III) with Charlotte Carolina screw and bone marrow aspirate concentrate: an outcome study in athletes. Am J Sports Med 2011; 39(6): 1295-301.
[http://dx.doi.org/10.1177/0363546510393306] [PMID: 21212308]

[12]   O'Malley M, DeSandis B, Allen A, Levitsky M, O'Malley Q, Williams R. Operative treatment of fifth metatarsal jones fractures (zones II and III) in the NBA. Foot Ankle Int 2016; 37(5): 488-500.
[http://dx.doi.org/10.1177/1071100715625290] [PMID: 26781131]

[13]   Hernigou P, Guissou I, Homma Y, *et al.* Percutaneous injection of bone marrow mesenchymal stem cells for ankle non-unions decreases complications in patients with diabetes. Int Orthop 2015; 39(8): 1639-43.
[http://dx.doi.org/10.1007/s00264-015-2738-2] [PMID: 25795249]

[14]   Adams SB, Lewis JS Jr, Gupta AK, Parekh SG, Miller SD, Schon LC. Cannulated screw delivery of bone marrow aspirate concentrate to a stress fracture nonunion: technique tip. Foot Ankle Int 2013; 34(5): 740-4.
[http://dx.doi.org/10.1177/1071100713478918] [PMID: 23463778]

CHAPTER 13

Risks of Bone Marrow Aspirate Concentrate

Benjamin David* and **Kevin Newman**

Ashford and St Peter's NHS Hospital, Surrey, UK

Abstract: The uses of expanded stem cells and BMAC have always been linked with potential concerns. The aim of this chapter is to highlight the potential concerns that have been reported in the available literature.

Keywords: Bone Marrow, Bone Marrow Aspirate Concentrate (BMAC), Complications, Stem Cells.

INTRODUCTION

The uses of bone marrow aspirate concentrate (BMAC) are widespread in medicine with further uses being continually developed. In the field of orthopaedics, their use includes aiding fracture healing, treatment of non-union and treatment of degenerative disease amongst many others. The use of BMAC, however, is not without risk. These can be divided into those occurring during the harvest of bone marrow and during the administration of the centrifuged product.

HARVEST

Bleeding

Whilst a relatively recent treatment in orthopaedics, the role of bone marrow aspiration to aid the diagnosis and treatment of haematological malignancies is well established. Many studies have been undertaken by haematologists to identify those patients at risk of bleeding intra- and post procedure. One of the largest studies involved almost 20,000 patients and only 11 of these experienced significant haemorrhage [1]. From this study, the most significant risk factors were found to be; current or recent anticoagulant therapy using agents including aspirin, warfarin and heparin; renal failure and a diagnosis of myeloproliferative disorder.

---

* **Corresponding author Benjamin David:** Ashford and St Peter's NHS hospital, Surrey, UK; E-mail: BenDavid@Doctors.org.uk

Mohamed A Imam and Martyn Snow (Eds.)

Though not an independent risk factor, it is recommended that in patients with potentially difficult access to the harvest site (in the case of iliac crest harvest) and obese subjects, the use of computed tomography control should be considered [2].

Various sites in the body can be used for aspiration with each site exposing different potential vascular structures to the risk of injury. The only reported death from haemorrhage following BMAC aspiration was attributed to a retroperitoneal haemorrhage caused during iliac crest aspiration [3]. In such instances, prompt diagnosis is essential and where available, selective arterial embolisation should be undertaken.

Infection

It is less common than haemorrhage. Of the 19,259 procedures recorded in 2003, only 2 subjects reported problems with localised infection from the harvest site and both cases reported successful treatment with antibiotics [1]. The literature does not support prophylactic antibiotics for the harvest of bone marrow aspirate alone, however, this procedure is commonly combined with the administration of BMAC and in the presence of prolonged instrumentation and/or implantation of prostheses or metalwork, antimicrobial prophylaxis is more routinely administered.

Chronic Pain

Although dependent on the site of harvest, chronic pain can be experienced followed by aspiration. The mechanism behind chronic pain is poorly understood but in refractory cases that do not spontaneously resolve, neuropathic pain medications may be of use. Of the 20,000 aspirates taken in 2003, only 2 subjects reported pain lasting more than several weeks [4].

In bone of low density, fractures must also be considered. Common sites of harvest include the iliac crest, tibia and femur. Studies have shown, however, that the highest yield of mesenchymal stem cells (MSCs) and most significant clinical outcomes come from the iliac crest aspiration [5].

In view of this being the commonest site of harvest and the risks of peritoneal and neurovascular damage with incorrect trocar placement, much work has been written regarding the ideal placement of the trocar. One such method involves dividing the iliac crest into quadrants, as devised by Hernigou *et al.* and previously described within this book [6].

ADMINISTRATION

Infection

If used as a sole treatment, most authors do not advocate prophylactic antimicrobial therapy, however, in the presence of prostheses such as in non union surgery, prophylaxis is routinely administered [7, 8]. The risks of infection from BMAC therapy are common to all surgical site infections (SSIs) and routine universal aseptic precautions should be used.

Fat Embolization

When applied intraosseously, due to the bone remaining permeable to the liquefied material, fat embolisation is a likely prospect [9]. Animal studies have explicated fat particles in dogs' lungs post-mortem [10], nonetheless in human trials, unfavourable clinical outcomes in the pattern of respiratory complications or reduced oxygen saturation have not been promulgated. Those subjects are at a higher hazard of embolization such as those with cardiac shunts should be examined as to their appropriateness to receive intraosseous BMAC. In all cases of intraosseous administration, patients should be observed for the clinical manifestations of fat embolism.

Risk of Tumorigenesis

One of the biggest anxieties with the application of BMAC into a distinct location is the potential risk for tumorigenesis. Nonetheless, this hypothesis is unproven in a large cohort by Hernigou *et al.* [11]. Over sixteen years, they retrospectively examined 1873 patients treated with BMAC at an average follow-up of 12.5 years. Patients were monitored for the existence of cancer from the time of the initial surgery continuously till death. They examine more than 7300 MRIs and 52,000 radiographs and reported the diagnosis of malignancy in 53 cases. All the 53 diagnoses of cancers were reported in areas other than the BMAC injection site. But, as per the recorded frequency of cancer in the general community, the contemplated incidence over the corresponding study time period was apparently between 97 and 108. This study observed no elevated cancer risk in cases after the application of BMAC either at the treatment site or elsewhere in 1873 after a mean follow-up period of 12.5 years.

CONSENT FOR PUBLICATION

Not applicable.

CONFLICT OF INTEREST

The authors declare no conflict of interest, financial or otherwise.

ACKNOWLEDGEMENTS

Declared none.

REFERENCES

[1]   Bain BJ. Bone marrow biopsy morbidity: review of 2003. J Clin Pathol 2005; 58(4): 406-8.
       [http://dx.doi.org/10.1136/jcp.2004.022178] [PMID: 15790706]

[2]   Devaliaf V, Tudor G. Bone marrow examination in obese patients. Br J Haematol 2004; 125(4): 538-9.
       [http://dx.doi.org/10.1111/j.1365-2141.2004.04936.x] [PMID: 15142126]

[3]   Arellano-Rodrigo E, Real MI, Muntañola A, *et al.* Successful treatment by selective arterial
       embolization of severe retroperitoneal hemorrhage secondary to bone marrow biopsy in post-
       polycythemic myelofibrosis. Ann Hematol 2004; 83(1): 67-70.
       [http://dx.doi.org/10.1007/s00277-003-0683-4] [PMID: 14574461]

[4]   Bain BJ. Bone marrow biopsy morbidity and mortality. Br J Haematol 2003; 121(6): 949-51.
       [http://dx.doi.org/10.1046/j.1365-2141.2003.04329.x] [PMID: 12786808]

[5]   Hauser RA, Orlofsky A. Regenerative injection therapy with whole bone marrow aspirate for
       degenerative joint disease: a case series. Clin Med Insights Arthritis Musculoskelet Disord 2013; 6:
       65-72.
       [http://dx.doi.org/10.4137/CMAMD.S10951] [PMID: 24046512]

[6]   Hernigou P. Understanding bone safety zones during bone marrow aspiration from the iliac crest: the
       sector rule Int ortho 2014; 38(11): 2377-2384
       [http://dx.doi.org/10.1007/s00264-014-2343-9]

[7]   Nejadnik H, Hui JH, Feng Choong EP, Tai BC, Lee EH. Autologous bone marrow-derived
       mesenchymal stem cells *versus* autologous chondrocyte implantation: an observational cohort study.
       Am J Sports Med 2010; 38(6): 1110-6.
       [http://dx.doi.org/10.1177/0363546509359067] [PMID: 20392971]

[8]   Kon E, Buda R, Filardo G, *et al.* Platelet-rich plasma: intra-articular knee injections produced
       favorable results on degenerative cartilage lesions. Knee Surg Sports Traumatol Arthrosc 2010; 18(4):
       472-9.
       [http://dx.doi.org/10.1007/s00167-009-0940-8] [PMID: 19838676]

[9]   Husebye EE, Lyberg T, Røise O. Bone marrow fat in the circulation: clinical entities and
       pathophysiological mechanisms. Injury 2006; 37 (Suppl. 4): S8-S18.
       [http://dx.doi.org/10.1016/j.injury.2006.08.036] [PMID: 16990064]

[10]   Orlowski JP, Julius CJ, Petras RE, Porembka DT, Gallagher JM. The safety of intraosseous infusions:
       risks of fat and bone marrow emboli to the lungs. Ann Emerg Med 1989; 18(10): 1062-7.
       [http://dx.doi.org/10.1016/S0196-0644(89)80932-1] [PMID: 2802282]

[11]   Hernigou P, Homma Y, Flouzat-Lachaniette CH, Poignard A, Chevallier N, Rouard H. Cancer risk is
       not increased in patients treated for orthopaedic diseases with autologous bone marrow cell
       concentrate. J Bone Joint Surg Am 2013; 95(24): 2215-21.
       [http://dx.doi.org/10.2106/JBJS.M.00261] [PMID: 24352775]

SUBJECT INDEX

A

Adipose tissues 7, 9, 10, 61, 65
Adjunctive treatment 75, 76
Adult bone marrow 82, 83
Adult human bone marrow cells 7
Adult tissues 7, 23
Advanced therapy medicinal product
    (ATMPs) 29
American spinal injury Association (ASIA) 84
Anabolic 60
Ankle fracture nonunions 106
Ankle surgery 104, 105, 106
Arthroscopic repair groups 71
Articular cartilage 68, 69, 70, 71
ASIA scale 84
Aspiration 10, 13, 52, 90, 92, 109
Autogenous BMAC 91
Autologous BMAC 71, 92
Autologous chondrocyte implantation (ACI)
    70, 71, 72
Autologous MSCs 25, 63
Avascular necrosis 75
Axonal regeneration 81, 82

B

Bilateral tibial 53, 55
Biological materials 30, 51, 52
Biomechanical characteristics 97
BMAC application 54, 76
BMAC group 71, 76, 105, 106
BMAC in foot and ankle surgery 104, 105,
    106
BMAC injection 52, 76, 99, 100
BMSCs therapy 85
BMSCs transplantation 83, 84, 85
Bone 2, 5, 64, 75
  iliac 2, 5, 64
  trabecular 5, 75
Bone defects 13, 51, 53, 55
Bone formation 14, 105

Bone grafting 92
Bone healing 11, 13, 46, 53, 57, 104, 105
Bone marrow 1, 2, 5, 6, 7, 12, 22, 52, 60, 61,
    62, 64, 65, 68, 69, 75, 76, 77, 82, 83, 90,
    92, 96, 104, 108
Bone marrow aspirate 2, 5, 6, 11, 12, 51, 52,
    80, 82, 83, 91, 92, 108, 109
Bone marrow aspirate cells 22, 24
Bone marrow cells 7, 83
  isolated 83
  removed 7
Bone marrow harvest 6, 108
Bone morphogenetic protein (BMP) 51, 52,
    60, 104
Bone regeneration 24, 45, 52, 53, 54, 55, 56
Buffy coat layer 98

C

Calcaneus 2, 6
Calcified zone 69
Cartilage defects 68, 70
Cartilage regeneration 63, 71
Cell-based therapy 23, 30
Cell death 75
Cells/million-nucleated cells 1
Cell therapy 29, 80, 81
Cellular elements 12
Cellular therapy 7, 8
Centrifugation 2, 11, 12, 14, 70
Chondrocytes 14, 68, 70, 76
Chondrogenic 61, 63
Clear benefits 68, 70
Clinical applications 5, 6, 7, 11, 69
Clinical implications of expanded stem cells
    61
Clinical trial authorization 29
Clinical trial data sharing 37, 49
Clinical trial design 36, 42, 46
Clinical trial endpoints 37
Clinical trial environment 47
Clinical trial reporting 37

www.ingramcontent.com/pod-product-compliance
Lightning Source LLC
Chambersburg PA
CBHW041716210326

41598CB00007B/675